A Psychoanalysis Influenced by Dissidence, Decoloniality, and Feminism

A Psychoanalysis Influenced by Dissidence, Decoloniality, and Feminism analyzes the intersection of psychoanalysis with feminisms, decolonial theories, philosophy and queer theory.

Fernando Barrios asks key questions such as: Is psychoanalysis a Eurocentric invention based on a colonial logos, and is there room for anything else? What can psychoanalysis say about the racialisation of bodies, poverty, and class? What can it say not only about the subjective effects of systems of oppression but also about the very production of subjectivity within them? Barrios considers texts and authors who rarely meet in dialogue – Indigenous, Chicano, and border feminisms, Jean Genet and authors of the anti-social turn in the queer field, Sigmund Freud and Jacques Lacan in tension with Monique Wittig and Judith Halberstam, Paul B. Preciado and Isabelle Stengers, Donna Haraway and Bruno Latour, the ontological turn and the affective turn – generating a field of productive tension. Through these cross-readings, the book examines the effects of a psychoanalysis that allows itself to be affected by contemporary discourses and practices in a situated manner.

A Psychoanalysis Influenced by Dissidence, Decoloniality, and Feminism will be of great interest to psychoanalysts in practice and in training, and to academics and scholars of psychoanalytic and Lacanian studies, feminisms, queer theory, critical theory, and decolonial theories.

Fernando Barrios is a psychoanalyst and member of the École Lacanienne de Psychanalyse. He coordinates the working group Zona Degenerada and is a member of the editorial committee for the digital platform e-dicciones Justine. An artist and curator, he is a member of the staff of the Contemporary Art Foundation (FAC) in Uruguay.

A Psychoanalysis Influenced by Dissidence, Decoloniality, and Feminism

De/Generating Psychoanalysis

Fernando Barrios

Routledge
Taylor & Francis Group
LONDON AND NEW YORK

Designed cover image: © Getty Images

First published in English 2026
by Routledge
4 Park Square, Milton Park, Abingdon, Oxon OX14 4RN

and by Routledge
605 Third Avenue, New York, NY 10158

Routledge is an imprint of the Taylor & Francis Group, an informa business

Translated by DeepL

Published in Spanish as *De/generar psicoanálisis* by Witz editor 2023

A catalogue record for this book is available from the British Library

ISBN: 978-1-041-19150-6 (hbk)
ISBN: 978-1-041-19149-0 (pbk)
ISBN: 978-1-003-71029-5 (ebk)

DOI: 10.4324/9781003710295

Typeset in Times New Roman
by Apex CoVantage, LLC

To the dead who accompany me from a thriving and encouraging spectrality and who I imagine laugh a lot at my sleeplessness.

To myself for not ceasing to be inconsistent and doing something about it.

Contents

Acknowledgements

To Julieta Lopérgolo, without whom this book would not exist. To my friends and colleagues at the École Lacanienne de Psychanalyse, who made me think that another psychoanalysis is possible. To each of the publishers and virtual sites that received these articles at their origin. To e-dictions justine for being one of the spaces in which I write. To Café y psicoanálisis and Tribu, a space that we support with José Assandri and in which some of these notions were conceived. To Sandra Filippini, companion of more than one writing adventure. To Zona degenerada, a collective of cross-readings that for years has been affecting me and producing me as a subject of discourse. To the Fundación de Arte Contemporáneo and especially to Fernando López Lage, who is a lucid interlocutor of ideas and an actor who helps me to bring some of this into the field of art. To Laura Falcón, friend and sister in life who puts up with this sometimes difficult to bear intensity that I am. To my analyst, who knew how to live through a transference that was sometimes hard, always critical, and was able to read the effect of the wounds that constitute me. To Jorge Reitter and Thamy Ayouch, friends whom I admire and love, with whom I imagine we sometimes recreate some version of Otras Yeguas del Apocalipsis. To Vero A. Cardozo and Jesica Ramírez, who received me in La tercera as immemorial friends, barely knowing me. To Lina Rovira, with whom we have shared multiple affections since we met. To Witz editor, to Guillermo Giménez and Veco – who did the cover design – and who thought it was desirable to run the risk of publishing these dissimilar texts, testimony of a journey, rather than a standard academic or essayistic book. To my family, who I suppose must have often wished that I had dedicated myself to the theatre – which I could have done – but who know how to hide it and love me. To all the authors who have marked this practice of saying what one knows is finally impossible and yet . . .

Introduction

De/generating psychoanalysis examines the effects of a psychoanalysis that allows itself to be affected by contemporary discourses and practices in a situated manner. Feminisms, queer theory, decolonial theories, as well as contributions from Michel Foucault, Deleuze, and Gauttari, among others, are critically assembled, generating a field of productive tensions. *De/generar* alludes both to the degenerate as a queer appropriation of a nosological category that has become an insult and to distancing itself from the sex-gender system that underlies the dominant heteronormativity to which psychoanalysis has inadvertently contributed. This movement of importunity and affectation is carried out situately, that is, from the geopolitical implication of a global south that seeks a non-Eurocentric analytic discourse, a *sud/acá.*

This book is something of a collage and a montage, articulating presentations and texts produced for different occasions and events that nonetheless multiply their effects by exploring the biases of cross-readings of authors who rarely meet in dialogue: Indigenous, Chicano, and border feminisms, Jean Genet and authors of the anti-social turn in the queer field, Sigmund Freud and Jacques Lacan in tension with Monique Wittig and Jack Halberstam, Paul B. Preciado and Isabelle Stengers, Donna Haraway and Bruno Latour, the ontological turn and the affective turn, and much more. Therefore, one should not expect a single thesis to guide the entire book, but rather a device for intervening in psychoanalysis that repositions it in contemporary conversation. Added to this is the fact that the writer situates her speech, situates her enunciation from her own subjective implication, making her own the feminist wager: the personal is political, and doubling down on the wager: the singular is political.

Prologue

Jorge N. Reitter

Promenade – Note on De/Generating Psychoanalysis

In August 1873, Viktor Hartmann, the Russian architect, painter, and sculptor, died of an aneurysm at the age of 42. A posthumous exhibition of his paintings was organised, and his close friend (I like to think of them as very close) Modest Mussorgsky wrote a suite for piano entitled *Pictures at an Exhibition*. In 1922, Maurice Ravel would orchestrate it magnificently. The different numbers of the suite musically depict some of the paintings of the exhibition, which are linked by the theme *promenade, promenade*. Mussorgsky accompanies us on a stroll through the exhibition and comments on his impressions of some of the paintings.

In the Mussorgsky manner, I will invite you to accompany me on my promenade through the texts of this book, which stands out for the quality of the writing in the often disappointing universe of psychoanalytic literature. This corresponds to my own promenade, as I read the book while on pilgrimage to places to which I was returning after a two-year wait, pandemic or no pandemic. So it was that I read it in the Villa Borghese in Rome, in a square whose name I don't know in Orvieto, in the Parc de Belleville, in that beautiful little square where Île Saint Louis ends, a lot in the Place des Vosges, which was my neighbourhood square for two weeks, and in Chueca, the most queer/degenerate of neighbourhoods.

Rather arbitrarily, I tend to separate writers into those who go the way of Proust and those who go the way of Joyce. In that personal taxonomy, I have Fernando Barrios clearly placed on the Joyce side, and in this way I am thinking of Fernando as a writer. I don't know if he was a psychoanalyst before, but at least at the same time as a psychoanalyst. It must be said, it is very rare to find in psychoanalytic literature a prose so original, so beautiful, and in which form and content, idea and words, are so successfully articulated. Fernando has that Joycean, but also Lacanian, talent for playing with words, for twisting them, re-twisting them so that they produce an unexpected and illuminating meaning, sometimes even funny.

Fernando does not write "Degenerar psicoanálisis", but "De/generar psicoanálisis", and that slash changes everything, multiplies the meanings. Translating or transforming *queer* into degenerate seems to me to be a formidable success, because it gives back to the word, in a Spanish-speaking context, the power of abjection that is lost in a word, *queer*, which in our milieu can sound rather *cool*. "Something of the subjective constitution does not take place in the same way everywhere; something of the experience of bodies in relation to a land and a language, to a symbolic, an imaginary and a real are not outside objective and subjective conditions of existence".

Fernando is radical, in the sense that he can sustain that almost impossible asceticism that is a queer position. When I read him, I have the impression that he would propose that we burn everything and start over from scratch, that we don't rescue anything from the past because it is always contaminated by too many things. He says it himself: "something in me leads me to adhere – why deny it – to an antisocial, anti-communitarian, anti-dentitarian radicalism, etc.". This is a position that I would never be able to sustain; it is beyond my strength. That is why reading him is always attractive and stimulating for me, and these differences do not hinder dialogue or friendship, on the contrary.

Fernando's book seeks, in the manner of Socrates-Tabanus, to annoy psychoanalysis (in that we are similar). Not out of a pure desire to fuck around, to *épater le bourgeois*, but to renew, so as not to become stagnant, so that psychoanalysis recovers the edge that it can so easily lose. So that we don't stop thinking. Take note that today feminisms, queer theory, and the decolonial are bothering psychoanalysis, which would be fine, except that a certain psychoanalysis doesn't want to be bothered. A certain psychoanalysis wants to be left alone to sleep, or not to be bothered by pickets when it wants to get to *the country*. Fernando writes:

> But what are the things that psychoanalysis is bothered about? The answer is so simple as to be absurd: everything. And surely some Lacanian will not remind me of Lacan's not everything, *pas tout*, so I will sharpen my aim: psychoanalysis is bothered in its not-everything. Not because it is necessary to take up some kind of totality – quite the contrary – but because perhaps it is time to review how not-all this not-all is, if it excludes exclusions that constitute and institute it.

I wish I could write with such elegance and such precision. In another passage, he says it in a way that I find particularly beautiful:

> It is not about a politics of cancellation but about an astonished re-reading of the inadvertencies and slips, of a critical and self-critical look at and from psychoanalysis as discourse and situated practice, politics and matrix of subjectivation, from the setting in tension and the crossing with other discursivities.

I think I recognise someone who is in the position of an analyst, something that has nothing to do with reciting paragraphs from some seminar of Lacan, but in being able to write sentences like this: "There is also an *unresolved* tension between a saying of the jouissance that causes us, and a not wanting to know anything about that jouissance" (italics are mine).

Fernando states that:

> If there is an ethic of writing in psychoanalysis, it is that of writing only about what concerns us, involves us, constitutes us. It is not a question of prescribing *coming out*, which would be a contradiction in terms, but of wanting a certain warning that it is not possible to speak except from ourselves, that is, from this fabulation of identity, this somatopolitical fiction that we are and that we perform.

Since he loves radical positions, he takes the pro: "And by the way, its flipside, not to speak of others, about others, for others . . .". But these differences matter little, because what counts is that this book is coherent with the ethics it proposes; therefore, it is a book that, while not at all simple in its proposals, I find easy to read. Easy insofar as the author's voice, which does not hide in any supposed neutrality, permanently summons us. One of those books that we don't want to put down.

I would like to conclude this *promenade* by giving the floor to Fernando, in a few paragraphs where he summarises what in my opinion is the most essential part of the book's theoretical, political. and ethical commitment:

> For a long time we subaltern subjects have been talked about, theorised, objectified and subjectified by others who, from positions of privilege, thought it necessary to highlight the deviation from the normal in order to make the exceptions the justification for the rule.
>
> Today we are spoken about by others, often from a paternalistic point of view. However, for some time now, we montruxs have been taking the floor, and I don't believe that we will be silenced, or that we will be silenced.
>
> Return of the oppressed.

Chapter 1

Degenerate

De/generate

I always knew of the eccentric, of the mismatch, of the non-coincidence, of the contradiction, of the impossibility of convincing myself of anything, of the suspicion about everything, of an irrevocable intention to twist everything, to un-twist everything, to turn me around like a sock, to put me on the opposite side of the agreement, of the asphyxiation of any us, of the possibility that we inhabit parallel worlds only imaginary united by the same language? that nothing guarantees more than equivocation, of the constitutive strangeness of everything and of myself, that there are nothing but beautiful monsters dressed in ugly normalities, that the exception is the rule and that we know it and we don't say it . . . we won't say it.

> *What I won't say.*
>
> (Alliance Francaise de Montevideo Exhibition, 2020)

From an (im)possible queer camp

Some time ago I wrote:

> To posit something like the existence of a *field* may entail the slippage or imaginary drift of something unified, coherent or consistent. Nothing could be further from the point we are trying to make. Firstly, because there is a logical-linguistic impediment in uniting in this way the rare, the strange, the a-normal and an order, a substantialisation or unity or politics of identity.
>
> (Barrios, 2017b, p. 2)

Nevertheless, something insists on the register of a certain (im)possibility.

I also said on that occasion that "political effects do not always subscribe to discursive logics and so, even in the interests of the market, it could be possible to enunciate: *¡todxs queer!*" (Barrios, 2017b). *Todxs queer*, *nadie queer* . . . in the logic of an inclusion that is as politically correct as it is problematic. Because even inclusion – I am playing with redundancy – is in question.

DOI: 10.4324/9781003710295-1

First, I would like to point out that, in my opinion, the debt to *feminisms* – as well as to *gay and lesbian studies* – is something not to be neglected (with the exception of feminism that ignores or openly rejects trans issues; such is the case of terfs – trans-exclusionary radical feminists, who see trans women as an abominable parody or as a Frankenstein phenomenon, techno-phallocratic, etc.).

From the assertion: *there is no queer theory without feminisms*, and including all activisms (gay, lesbian, trans, intersex, etc.) and the production of texts and visuals, through the rupture in the consideration of the *bi-woman* as a political subject, to trans-feminism and its expansion and rupture with all identity essentialism of the so-called feminine, I do not believe that an insoluble separation of fields is possible or desirable, but rather a putting in tension, a putting theoretical productions and micro-political activisms and practices to work together. Likewise, Jack Halberstam's (2015) warning about the need for multiple genealogies and not to stick to one "heroic archive" seems more than tenable.

If it is a question of tracing the so-called *queer theory* from its beginnings to the present day, pointing out biases, open lines, turns, in very diverse authors: Judith Butler, Gayle Rubin, Paul B. Preciado, J. Halberstam, D. Halperin, Leo Bersani, Lee Edelman, Heather Love, Gloria Anzaldúa, and many others, it is necessary to ask oneself: What are the consequences and effects of dissent from heteronormativity in the fields of thought, art and psychoanalysis, among others, and in the lives of all?

The term *queer theory* was coined by Teresa de Lauretis, in 1991, as:

> a critical project aimed at undoing or resisting the cultural and sexual homogenisation in academia of so-called "lesbian and gay" studies, which was seen as a single field of research. But, of course, this was not the case: gay men and lesbians had different histories, different ways of relating to each other and different sexual practices. Lesbians were not, at that time, the main targets of gay "lifestyle" marketing strategies (round-the-clock saunas, cruises and package holidays, fashion). Moreover, lesbians had a strong, if sometimes conflicting, relationship with the feminist movement. Indeed, issues of racial and ethnic difference, raised by black, Chicana and Latina lesbian collectives in their critique of white feminism, were to shape feminism in the 1980s and beyond.

My interest, for some time now, together with others, has been to work on queer theory – Lacanian psychoanalysis – contemporary art and other practices derived from sexual dissidence from heteronormativity. In order to do so, I believe it is necessary to reference the points, the drifts, the biases that question the queer field today.

Let us begin with queer as a *word* and as a *category*. As a word it tells us nothing in Spanish, that is to say, something does not pass into Spanish. On some occasions we have asked ourselves whether it would be *degeneradx* an alternative. This is no minor matter; the appropriation of an insult, and the attempt to do something else with it has had and has consequences for those who embark on this appropriationist and performative act.

As *a category*, it runs the risk – as we pointed out earlier – of producing the illusion of consistency, of grouping – which is always in-grouping[1] – of unifying the diverse. And beyond the fact that it is a logical impossibility, queer is the opposite of all universalisation, categorisation, etc. I don't think it is convenient to fall into political naivete: everything can be reabsorbed by a voracious symbolic that always includes, normalises, neutralises, deproblematises.

Second, there is the question of *language*: how to say what is different, what is non-heteronormative in our language. I am no longer referring to its nomination but to its writing and the practices of saying. Orality, writing, and images will be planes on which other modes of non-representation will operate. There is a need to operate in language or to allow ourselves to be operated by another language that tries to say the other, through neologisms or turns of phrase, liberating language from a sexual politics that is always sexist. We could rephrase Gayatri Spivac's (2003) now canonical question: can the subaltern speak? How can subalternity speak? How can the subaltern be said?

Already Lacan (1972–1973) coined the term *lalangue*, all together to account for the singularity of the relationship of each subject-subject to the language. And poets and artists have always done something else with language(s). There is a relation to language to be checked in each one of us.

A third point that arises for me – as an artist and curator – is: what *images* for the degenerate[2] is it possible to speak of contemporary and degenerate art in our (local and regional) art scene? It is certainly not a question of making the degenerate an adjective; it could only be justified if we do so as a provocation. It is rather, perhaps, to allow ourselves to be pierced by a queer-decolonial-dissident warning, and so on.

The so-called *decolonial turn* is then another issue to be debated in this archaeology of the contemporary: what are the consequences for our practices (analytical, artistic, among others) of the works of Anibal Quijano, Walter Mignolo, Rita Segato, as well as those of Silvia Rivera Cusicanqui, or further back in time of Rodolfo Kush and his problematisation of being/being? More recently, these demarcations have been taken up again by Paola Arboleda Ríos (2011) in "Ser o estar queer en Latinoamérica" and by the whole field of so-called decolonial aesthetics.

The contribution of *black feminisms*: Ochi Curiel, Audre Lorde, and mestizos with Gloria Anzaldúa, lesbian, Chicana and mestizo, and others, make us continue to think about how it is possible to account for the *colonial heritage*.

Another shift or bias is the so-called *anti-social turn*, which questions the goodness and benefits of inclusion, from Leo Bersani (1998) in *Homos*, fundamentally in the chapter "The gay before the law", or from the readings of Didier Eribon (2004) on Jean Genet or more recently Lee Edelman (2014) with *No Future*. What are the costs of being accepted, tolerated, admitted as citizens, as equals?

Perhaps one of the greatest exponents of this turn is precisely Lee Edelman, who proposes to stop sustaining *reproductive futurism*, to make ourselves flesh of the death drive, to become *synthomosexual* (a neologism created from Lacan's neologism), to abandon the figure of the child as the figure of the future, the taboo horizon of all politics. Reproductive futurism is redundant for the discursive logic of this author, insofar as all futurism is reproductive. Thus, even *desire* itself – although I think here more in the Freudian notion of desire – is called into question insofar as it points to something that is on the horizon of a future, of something to come. The future of an illusion?

Already Leo Bersani in the above-mentioned chapter challenged his readers: "Should a homosexual be a good citizen?" re-affirming the "furore over the respectability" of gays and lesbians in the struggle for civil rights – including marriage – and clarifying that "there is no doubt that we must defend the rights of people to adhend whatever worthy or unworthy cause inspires them". André Gide, in *The Immoralist*, points out through the mouth of his protagonist Michel:

> only naked figure . . . remove and if homosexuality is somehow linked to that nakedness, with its longing for the *delicious company of the dregs of society*, and the anguished need to free itself from its fortuna, then we must take a closer look at this curious sexual preference which seems to demand the repudiation of property and a renunciation of citizenship.

The notion of a "non-relational pederasty" could be one of the precursors of this anti-social turn I am referring to. Particularly since from Jean Genet and the ethical demand of *betrayal* in a particular *asceticism* in "a defiant refusal of the codes of mourning". This could hardly leave psychoanalysis untouched, if we are willing to be problematised.

For their part, from the so-called affective turn, authors such as Heather Love and Carolyn Dinshaw resituate affect. For the authors of the affective turn, "the emotional, sentimental and even erotic dimension of the relationship between the past and the present appears as an unavoidable element when it comes to creating alternative historical narratives about dissident sexuality" (Dinshaw, 1999).

It is not only a matter of integrating the affects experienced by the subjects of history, but also of a subjective position of the person who researches, studies, or reads, which does not avoid the *bodily-affective* experience, which does not avoid "affecting" itself in this connection with the past. Perhaps the figure of Michel Foucault when he says in *La vie des hommes infamilles (The Lives of Infamous Men)* – I can't help but notice that he says men – that he had a physical sensation while researching. As Mariela Solana (2016) points out:

> Foucault speaks of a "vibration" he felt while studying those singular and abject lives of the past and how the fragments he found caused him a physical impression and an intensity hardly passible to be reconstructed by means of historical writing.

For the medievalist historian Carolyn Dinshaw (1999), it is a matter of moving away from a triumphalist turn that masks the suffering of those who lived their sexual dissidence in times of greater discrimination and violence. It is not a question of returning to shame and guilt in order to go backwards, but to recover their critical potential. Those who point to the need to generate *archives of dissidence* in each country, in each city, are moving in the same direction. Something of making visible and processing what has been experienced, not in order to remain there but precisely to be able to move on to something else: "exploring its negative charge for the value it has in itself, for its capacity to tell us something about the experience of living with the injury", says H. Love (2007).

On the other hand, and in a very different way, and in tension with the above, there is someone like David Halperin and his idea of *the queer in the gay*, who denaturalises the "heterosexual dramaturgy of affects", or Javier Saez with his sentence "love is heterosexual", broadening and complicating the critical spectrum. It seems interesting to me to contrast the so-called affective turn with the critical positions of heteronormative affectivity proposed as universal.

Saez gives the queer field the slap in the face of *El amor es heterosexual*, and David Halperin brings back to the stage a cultural dimension of the gay – as *cultural practices* – where he locates the queer, proposing that the supposed hegemonic affectivity is nothing more than "a heterosexual dramaturgy of the affections", a political performance.

Saez (2015) states:

> I wonder if the rhetoric of love is just another discourse and another practice that we have adopted from the heterosexual regime. In any case, it is a totally harmless and domesticated discourse, something that does not bother the patriarchal and homophobic system at all. On the contrary, buns, queers and even transgender people are much better digested and accepted when they have a father ("what healthy boys, they are no longer promiscuous") and above all when they proclaim "their love" ("look how nice they are, they love each other; they are like us"). As Foucault said,
>
> what bothers power is not homosexual relations, but friendship. That is to say, the possibility of creating networks of friends, support, affection, solidarity, which are difficult to locate, which escape social control and which go beyond the individualist or liberal binary model: "couple-love-marriage". My impression is that love remains the last bastion that no one dares to cross, to question. It is presented as something universal, ahistorical, intrinsically good, human, positive. But perhaps there is no love in the singular, there is no love without history, there is no love without relations of power, class and race, perhaps one can live without love . . .". He concludes: "love is the master's tool. It was written, but we did not see it: love.

David Halperin, for his part, tries to resituate *the queer in gay*, no longer in sexual practices but in *cultural practices* and in a different *gaze*, deviant and defiant, subverting everything that is institutionalised, rarefying, queerising: "gay culture has a propensity to laugh at situations that are horrible or tragic in the eyes of others", he affirms. And he starts from this observation to resituate the de-generic or anti-generic game of gay and trans humour. And he exemplifies: "drag shows have canonised, preserved and renewed this tradition". Halperin inserts these manifestations within what he calls: "a gay cultural habitus, a deliberately anti-social aesthetic trajectory". It is a look and not a sexual practice. Fragments of straight culture taken out of context – and gendered, degenerated – take on deviant, other meanings. It seems clear to Halperin that gay culture and straight culture, regardless of the sexuality of those who embody it, engage in a different logic of gender.

The *heteronormative gaze* is described as: serious, categorical, judgmental, moralising, psychologising, literal. For example, taking a raunchy comedy and, instead of laughing, seeing it as a documentary that attempts to deal with serious psychological and social problems. There is thus work to be done in terms of a denaturalisation of this "heterosexual dramaturgy of affects", work from which psychoanalysis would do well not to be left out, I think.

Judith Butler (2006), from the notions of *vulnerability and recognition*, "liveable lives", *mourning, etc.*, situates us before the *ethical turn* in the queer field; a turn that is not unproblematic. In the last few years, particularly since the publication of *Precarious Life*, Butler points to the ethical reconfiguration of the political, understood in terms of relationships. It assigns a central place to the *vulnerability* to which every human being is confronted. We are politically constructed by virtue of the social vulnerability of our bodies. There is a condition of "initial dispossession": "we are handed over to the other from the outset, according to which from the very beginning, even prior to individuation itself and by virtue of our bodily existence, we are handed over to another". Violence impacts on this background of vulnerability.

However, the distribution of attention and care for this vulnerability is not the same for everyone, which is why it calls for "norms of recognition that sustain our persistence". What is needed then is "a process of 'cultural translation' in which language itself is broken and opened to the interpellation of other bodies and other languages; in which our most fundamental categories are dissolved and pushed to the limits of available epistemes".

The dissident erotics-psychoanalysis relation supposes an other edge, border, or terrain, riddled with tensions to (not) resolve. To cope, to accommodate, to let oneself be crossed, crossings, edges, points of friction, and non-submission of the fields. Jean Allouch and the question of the symptom in Lacan: what subject are we talking about; political subject/subject in Lacan/Foucault, subjectivities and agency in Deleuze and Guattari could be just the beginning of a list of complexities.

Lacan's "there is no sexual relation" ([1968–69] 2008a), as well as the notion that man and woman bear no other consistency than that of being signifiers, the non-mutuality of jouissance, nevertheless seem to enable some possible crossings.

Postporn, the inclusion of bodies with *functional diversity* and other bodies – "abject" for a heterosexual or hormone pornography – opens up other doors to the possibility of a new way of understanding the heteronormative pornography – opens other doors to dissident erotics and enables another visibility that is not without empowerment. Defined by Paul. B. Preciado (2014) as

> the process of becoming a subject of those bodies that until now had only been able to be abject objects of pornographic representation: women, sexual minorities, non-white bodies, transsexual, intersex and transgender people, deformed or disabled bodies. It is a process of empowerment and re-appropriation of sexual representation.

A new field of erotic visualities opens up to the gaze, just as the sadism-masochism (s/m) and the *erotics of violence* cease to be invisible or suspected of psychopathology, only gradually. Performances such as those of Bob Flanagan (Hart, 1998), who finds another way of dealing with the pain of his cystic fibrosis, or films such as *Crash* – in which jouissance is tied to the accident – and others, become critical epistemic supports of normativity.

From the *ecological turn*, ecofeminism and antispeciesism, other uprisings are taking place: "women and animals are not objects of patriarchal consumption" becomes a slogan. The speciesism of placing man as the superior species is seen as nothing more than the use of androcentric hegemony and its privileges. Richard Ryder, Stanley and Roslind Godlovitch, John Harris, or Peter Singer are just some of its representatives.

Authors such as Annie Sprinkle (2017), who defines herself as *ecosexual*, i.e., as someone who "is not afraid to have sexual relations with nature and/or technology". "We make love with the Earth through our senses", she says. The wager is on an "eco-logical erotic" practice, which does not hide the interdependence of a permeable and sensual self, from a desire for something "more than human", of which the human is only a part.

Intersexuality and the whole field of sexual variation disrupt biomedical certainties in a disruptive way. As Mauro Cabral (2005) points out: "we refer to all those situations in which the sexed body of an individual varies with respect to the culturally prevailing standard of feminine or masculine corporeality".

Variations range from:

> those involving chromosomal mosaics (xxy, xx0), particular configurations and locations of the gonads – (the coexistence of testicular and ovarian tissue, undescended testes) as well as of the genitalia (e.g., when the size of the penis is "too" small and when the clitoris is "too" large according to the same standard I spoke about before, when the end of the urethra is displaced, when the clitoris is "too" large according to the same standard I spoke about before, when the end of the urethra is displaced, when the size of the penis is "too" small and when the clitoris is "too" large according to the same standard mentioned above, when the end of the urethra is displaced from the tip of the penis to one of its sides or to the base of the penis, or when the vagina is absent).
>
> (Cabral, 2005)

For Cabral, this is "a very broad set of possible corporealities, whose variation with respect to 'typical' masculinity and corporeality is given by a cultural, biomedically specific way of looking at and measuring human bodies" (Cabral, 2005).

The *human* itself has been gaining and losing ground as a queer issue since its denaturalisation and de-universalisation. Authors such as Rosi Braidotti (2015) with *Lo posthumano* or Donna Haraway (1991) with *Manifiesto cyborg*, confront us with the limits of this notion.

Haraway says that in

> our age . . . a mythical time, we are all quimeras, theorised and fabricated hybrids of machine and organism; in short, we are cyborgs. This is our ontology, it gives us our politics. It is a condensed image of imagination and material reality, both centres which, united, structure any possibility of historical transformation.
> (1991)

Subversive virtuality is given by the fact that:

> The cyborg is decidedly on the side of partiality, irony, intimacy and perversity. It is oppositional, utopian and by no means innocent. Not being structured by the polarity of public and private, it defines a technological polis based partly on a revolution of social relations in the oikos, the family cell. Nature and culture are remodelled and the former can no longer be a resource to be appropriated and incorporated by the latter. The relationship to form toriums with parts, including those related to polarity and hierarchical domination, are paramount in the world of the cyborg.

Haraway opposes the cyborg to Frankenstein when she says:

> Unlike Frankenstein, the cyborg does not expect his father to save him by arranging the garden (of Eden), that is, by making a heterosexual couple, by finishing him off in a totality, in a city and in a cosmos. The cyborg does not dream of a community that follows the model of the organic family but without an oedipal project.

A new gauntlet thrown down to psychoanalysis, at least to a psychoanalysis that made the oedipus the guarantor of heteronormality.

Against the grain of Haraway, *Frankenstein* is, for a variety of people, a figure of the queer, of that which erases borders between genders and categories: dead-alive, body-pieces, human-non-human, nature-technology-culture, and so on.

For its part, the *monstrous* gains a place as dissidence; the monstrous as a place of abjection. Authors such as Atilio Raúl Rubino (1975) with "El monstruo *queer* en *The Rocky Horror Picture Show*. Sexualidad, género y parodia camp del cine de terror" ("The queer monster in *The Rocky Horror Picture Show.* Sexuality, gender and camp parody of horror cinema") show that "as a *camp* parody of horror cinema, it superimposes in the same body all the figures of monstrous otherness and makes them always signify sexuality and gender".

From Japanese *manga* animation and comics and *homoerotic anime*, particularly *Yaoi*, other non-Western visuals emerge that have a strong impact on the aesthetics and eroticisms of the masses of consumers who are growing day by day. Yaoi, as homoerotic pornography for women, is defined, according to Áurea Xaydé Esquivel Flores (2016), by:

> 1) the main characters are two: the *seme* (who "attacks") and the *uke* (who "receives"); in general, the personalities are opposite, so that the *seme* is usually older, quiet, sensual and dominant, while the *uke* is younger, loud, irritable and shy. Thus, 2) rape is a quasi-obligatory practice; since one refuses to reciprocate the other's feelings, the other is "forced" to show his or her love in a more overt way. 3) At the end of the story the relationship is affirmed, either in harmonious or conflicting terms, but the curious thing is that 4) the word or concept "gay" is rarely present, i.e., the gender of the loved one does not condition one's identity in any way, it just happens that a man's ideal partner turns out to be another man.

Lastly, and no less exempt from problems of different origins, the so-called *new masculinities* are making their appearance, with positions that range from a deliberate dis-marking of sex-generic privileges to betting on the de-essentialisation of the masculine, such as that of Judith Halberstam (2008) in *Masculinidad femenina (Female masculinity)*, for example.

In the first case, the so-called "men's groups", which at the academic and social level are grouped together to try to deconstruct the masculine from a greater or lesser degree of dis-marking, disidentification, with respect to patriarchal social mandates, without necessarily questioning the male-female binarism that is the basis of heteronormality. Another criticism of these groups is their refocusing on identity rather than on the power relations that underpin the sex-gender system. In the second case, *Judith* – today Jack – Halberstam.

He begins by asking: "If masculinity is not the social, cultural and political expression of virility, then what is it?", and affirms the illuminating value of the notion of *feminine masculinity* that "far from being an imitation of virility, . . . in reality, it gives us a clue as to how masculinity is constructed as such".

Halberstam is particularly attentive to the ideological implications or traversals at play in the staging of these masculinities. Thus, from the artistic field and the drag king performances, he proposes:

> Other attacks on dominant gender regimes come from performance and queer butch art, including drag king shows, butch theatre roles or art productions developed by genderqueer subjects. . . . Stars such as Elvis Herselvis or Mo B. Dick subvert dominant masculinity by making parodies of the superstar male and transforming conventional forms of sexism and misogyny into successful comedies. . . . Dick subverts dominant masculinity by making parodies of the

> superstar male and transforming conventional forms of sexism and misogyny into successful comedy. . . . Drag king Maureen Fischer succeeds in parodying masculinity by representing its most unnatural aspect and most often brought to the stage: sexism. By proclaiming to the public his heterosexuality, his fear of faggots and his desire for the "titis" in drag kings' clubs, Mo B. Dick reeks of misogyny. Mo B. Dick's manipulations of this staged theatrical masculinity look not only at the preformative aspect of masculinity, but also at the places where the non-preformative has ideological implications. In other words, by showing men's slimy approaches to women as theatrical, the drag king prevents any construction of misogyny as belonging to the natural order of things.

Gender ideology – and not gender ideology, in the sense in which the detractors of the queer field use this expression to delegitimise it – in the understanding that gender is in itself an ideological construction and a political regime – we have known this since Monique Wittig, at least – that seeks to order in a binary manner bodies and their enjoyments, which never cease to be ordered.

Surely there are many aspects or lines of flight left unmentioned in this mapping or thick sieve of what I consider to be the complexity today of a field that should not be neglected. So much for this kind of mapping or coarse sieve that surely does not exhaust, nor does it pretend to, the complexity of a field not to be neglected.

On the (non)future of a turn

"Of negativity in queer", "The anti-social turn in queer theory", or "The anti-social thesis in queer theory" would have been other possible names for this text; of course, the choice would not have been innocuous – as nothing is innocuous in the field of choices. However, something of an other-saying to which I submit, pleasantly and painfully, having dropped the remains of a university pretense, imposed itself.

One of the critiques that Judith, now Jack, Halberstam (2015) makes of Lee Edelman (2014), author of *No to the Future*, made an impact on me:

> Like Lacan and Virginia Woolf, and unlike the punks, he attempts to exercise obsessive control over the reception of his own discourse. Edelman's syntax, which twists, turns back on itself, and reveals the power of invention, shuts down the anarchy of meaning. In footnotes and other such formulations, Edelman closes himself off from criticism and hides the future and the fantasies of the future from the reader.
>
> Halberstam continues:
>
> predicts criticisms of his work for elitism, pretension, style and racism . . . etc. . . . having excluded the future, he continues on his way in a world of intelligence and chiasms closed in on himself. . . . He succumbs to the law of

grammar, the law of logic, the law of abstraction, the law of apolitical formalism and the law of genres.

Undoubtedly – though excessive – it seems to me to be a subtle and defiant critique for anyone who dares to write about *queer*, and why not, also about psychoanalysis, in psychoanalysis, in short. It also connects with an obsession of mine, with something that insists on what is written, on what it is to write, on what does not cease not to be written, on whether or not is anything written?

On the other hand, I confess at the outset, I feel much more attracted and challenged by Edelman's claim to (im)possible radicality. I also wonder whether gender and erotic determinants are not at play here. Although we may claim to be talking about the same thing, something about the experience of the history of the bodies that carry these sayings makes a difference. In fact – perhaps this is not just an anecdote – Teresa de Lauretis, who coined the term "queer theory", shortly after coining it, drops it and takes up the term *lesbian. Practices of Love*, her book from 1994, is proof of this.

Queer Theory emerged from the *Queer Theory* workshop organised in 1990 by de Lauretis "to resist cultural and sexual homogenisation in the academic field of gay and lesbian studies" and to rescue the differences within these collectives, differences that de Lauretis considered silenced. Racial and ethnic differences will be added to the differences between gays and lesbians, but the cooperative dialogue she hoped for will not happen.

As de Lauretis (2014) reminds us in a conference in Buenos Aires, just as we owe the notion of gender to feminist activism and not to academia – even though it was Gayle Rubin in 1975 who established the idea of the sex-gender system – we are indebted to gay activism in the appropriation of queer insult. In passing, I will say that for de Lauretis negativity is in the sexual, understood as the infantile, perverse-polymorphic, Freudian sexual, revisited by Jean Laplanche in his theory of generalised seduction. It is to think that it is Laplanche whom de Lauretis recognises as the introducer of gender in psychoanalysis.

Also in this brief visit to this author, I find very pertinent her idea that there is a need for reciprocal and successive translations between theory, politics, and sexual practices, something similar to what Gramsci did in the Marxist field. Otherwise, the confusion of fields makes some precision impossible.

My first approach to the subject came when I read Leo Bersani's *Homos* (1998), more precisely in chapter 4, "The outlaw gay". I am going to correct myself, because I should have said the first "intellectual" approach, because the opposite would be to maintain the illusion that one finds something that one had not already found in one's own life. The epiphany only produces its effects where it is expected.

I read *Homos* writing about Jean Genet, that is to say, in that shock that it meant for me to write using Genet. And if for Genet betrayal of the beloved is the greatest act of love, I hope I betrayed him well. Although I must surely have failed, and I regret it only a little, because I make Halberstam's idea that *queer* has to do with a certain art of failure my own. In an interview with Lucas Platero (2014), Halberstam says:

> In a society where success is defined in terms of capital accumulation and domesticity, *queer* people are relegated in both spheres to the space of failure, and in some ways, make failure a worthy project. In other words, to the extent that *queer* people want to disrupt social norms, they have to engage with failure, and as Samuel Beckett would say, "fail better".

David Halperin (2015), in *L'Art d'être gai*, on the subject of irony and gay humour, points to other renunciations: "by using one's own suffering in this way: as a vector of parody, one renounces sympathy, empathy, emotional consensus, identification, one sabotages the mechanisms of social discredit".

Some time ago I curated a show called *Degenerate Art*, and on that occasion there were many signs that I was exposing myself to some forms of discredit: a degenerated analyst? A curator posing for a photo-performance, in stockings, garter belts, and heels? A curator mingling with the artists? A show that takes an ironic look at the show that the Nazis made to discredit non-pure, non-Aryan art? Is it permissible to laugh at something so terrible? Is it permissible to laugh at something so terrible?

One of the artists performs a *drag queen* who rapes, "conchifies" objects with a penis-blade, visualising the very violence of gender assignment; doesn't this reproduce the violence that is being denounced, we were asked? Anti-social art? But what would a socially good art be? A useful, educational, edifying art?

Plato was clear: art is not involved in the education of virtuous citizens. And does psychoanalysis have a place in the city? Does the polis, the politics of the polis, admit a discourse and a practice that does not make a political bond? Undoubtedly, the question of the *social bond* – even if it is rarely mentioned – is one of the springs at play in the discussions about the convenience or inconvenience of the anti-social turn of the queer.

At a time of social and political conquests, of the expansion of rights and social services, of states opening up to protect minority groups, at a time of inclusion and normalisation, of happiness at last common to all, would it not be self-destructive to plead for a certain abnormality – in a very different sense from the one Joyce Mc Dougall gave it in her book *Plea for a Certain Abnormality* –, a desire to maintain and even claim *unintelligibility*, as Edelman and Bersani, and Genet without Sartre, do, non-absorption, abjection, non-futurity? "Apolitical negativity" is what Halberstam calls this position, which he calls risky, and he warns us of the "potentially sinister associations that can be made between apolitical negativity . . . and the masculinist anti-domestic and anti-reproductive politics of the homophile movements with Nazi tendencies of the early 1930s".

To this negativity, which he calls apolitical, he opposes as a wager a version of feminism that situates femininity in the negative territory of masochism, passivity, vulnerability and castration in artists such as Yoko Ono or Marina Abramovic, the negative freedom of Jamaica Kincaid, or the project of extermination of men of Valerie Solanas – although she does not seem to approve of their violence. Halberstam's critique also extends to the *archive* of Edelman or Bersani, which he calls "a heroic archive . . . composed of literary texts by Genet and other authors, rather than relying on the discouraging archive of texts on masculinist and transphobic anti-social sexism".

Nothing seems to me further from heroic than Jean Genet's living and writing journey, at least before the Sartrean rescue that almost killed him. There are loves that kill – there is no doubt about it. The title of this section of Halberstam's text makes sense to me at least: "Size does matter: small files" (Halperin, 2015). For someone who has written about female masculinities, this phallic slip does not seem minor. On the other hand, I agree, and his idea that "we need several genealogies of queer/lesbian/trans history" (Halperin, 2015) resonates very well with me, but not to be confined to the dimension of "political projects", but rather to make visible the different *relations to the political* and the social; the different ways of *being queer* and their impossibility of being.

Now then, let's look at some of what Lee Edelman (2014) plays with in *No to the Future*: *Queer theory and the death drive*, in his wager on negativity. A war machine book against *reproductive futurism*, that is, against all futurism. For Edelman, all bets on the future are based on the desire for social and personal reproduction, embodied in the figure of the Child. The child and his or her necessary protection as an unquestionable value of all politics. The political is such "to the extent that the fantasy underlying the image of the Child invariably shapes the logic by which the political itself must be thought of" (Edelman, 2014). And in this right and left go together:

> However radical the means by which certain voters try to produce a more desirable social order, it remains conservative at the centre because it is operating to affirm a structure, to authenticate a social order which it then tries to transmit to the future in the form of its inner Child.

The perpetual horizon of any policy, the future is the imperative "of enclosed in some stable and positive form". Politics is always positive, Halberstam will say, and de Lauretis and others will reiterate. It is in this sense that I do not think it is correct to say that Edelman's wager is apolitical; in any case it will be anti-political, counter-political, unless we play the *a* of the prefix not as a privative value but as an indication of a drift, a different relation to the political.

The possibility of constructing a non-teleological queer politics will certainly receive a negative response from Edelman. Politics is teleological or it is not politics. Let us add to this that in non-futurity there would be no possibility of a positive ethics that would ensure some supreme good. Lacan (2008b), in the seminar *Even*, which Edelman uses in the opening section of the book, refers to the sovereign good from which, he says, it has been thought possible to build an ethic. A sovereign good on which slippages have occurred over the course of time. It is in this sense that the queer achieves another ethical value, "more radical precisely insofar as it accesses this place, accepting its figurative status as a resistance to the viability of the social". A space unthinkable from the political, outside the perspective of a future, which Edelman links to the death drive as that which opposes all form, all gathering, all progress, all reproduction. And just as in the past activism had to appropriate what was originally an insult, an injury, now it will be time to appropriate what has been ejected, abjected, rejected from all politics, from all social projects – the place "of the death drive of the social order".

To paraphrase Javier Saez (2015) in "Love is heterosexual", I ask myself: is the social heterosexual? Heterosocial? The *queer* would point not to a good – whatever it may be – but to a "better", which Edelman links to Lacan's notion of truth, which aspires to the real (this is *Psychoanalysis, Radiophony and Television:* "I always tell the truth, not the whole truth, because we are not capable of telling the whole truth", Lacan, 1993). It is tempting to oppose this better to *O worse* (Lacan, 2012c), but it would be a facilism that I will not enable myself, that is to say, that I have already enabled.

Politics, Edelman adds, is based on the fantasy of a form, of an order that ensures identities, imaginary totalisations, goods, and satisfactions. It denies the hole in the Symbolic, its incompleteness. In this sense, politics in the Symbolic is a politics of the Symbolic. "Politics names that struggle to effect a phantasmatic order of reality where the alienation of the subject is vanished in a seamless identity at the end of that infinite chain of signifiers that has been lived as history".

"Politics is always a politics of the signifier", he says.

"It is a name for the temporisation of desire, for its translation into a narrative, for its teleological determination". In this there is a difference that appeared to me as interesting with respect to a statement by Jean Allouch (2013) to the effect that "To desire is to be without a future". It remains to be seen whether this still holds with the idea of *soulevement*, uprising or revolt, on which Allouch hovers today. For Edelman, on the contrary, desire always points to an unrealised, unrealisable future. The futureless future can only be accessed via the death drive and jouissance. The death drive as "inarticulable excess that dismantles the subject from within", so installed within the Symbolic, "by the loss of the Real that produces the advent of the signifier" (Edelman).

After Jean Allouch's seminar in Buenos Aires: *No heterosexual relation. heterosexual relation. Heterotic ii*, a question remained in my mind: is it really necessary to appeal to the death drive, or perhaps death itself, despite or precisely because of its unthinkable status, would do its negative work if we make room for it? Wouldn't death be operating those indomitable truths that Allouch extracts from the analytic exercise and the reading of Lacan? If sex and death are in solidarity, if language masks death and the sexual non-relation, would it not be death itself in its negative work, in the productive negativity of its work, that would allow these negative conquests? Wouldn't the freedom of the subject that Allouch proposes to bet on derive from a de-ended relation to death?

Some years ago, I wrote a little book of negative aphorisms, which I called *Desaforismos apócrifos y otras herjías (Apocryphal aphorisms and other heresies).* In a game of subversion of the popular wisdom that affirms that everything has a solution, one of them says: "The only thing that has a solution is death". I'm not even sure about that today anyway. At that point: sexual intercourse, God, future seem to produce something of a series.

Back to Edelman: "The only queerness that *queer* sexualities could aspire to signify would be born of their determined opposition . . . to the guiding fantasy according to which a symbolic closure will be achieved", finally realising the social subject. The possibility of radically dissolving the social-sexual contract that operates as a guarantee against the jouissance of the Real.

Guy le Gaufey recently recalled: "beware that when you listen to the real! – saying it with dramatic emphasis – *God is there*". In any case, Edelman clarifies: "it is not that we are, or can be, outside the Symbolic, but we can nevertheless choose to access our cultural production as figures – within the dominant logic of narrative, within symbolic reality – of the dismantling of that logic".

I will pause a little here. Throughout the reading of *No to the Future*, I couldn't help but ask myself, on what plane or enunciative level does what was being said there reside? That is to say, who is speaking? – although Beckett is not interested – and who is being spoken to?

Is it a manifesto? Because if so, I wouldn't have too much difficulty in adhering to it – even though I know that every manifesto presupposes another that will bring it down, and so on ad infinitum. That is to say, something in me leads me to adhere – why deny it? – to an anti-social, anti-communitarian, anti-dentitarian, etc. radicalism. However, if it is a question of each case, of each subject – if this formulation is viable – how can a certain subjective position be prescribed? What does it mean for any one person to figure or offer to figure the death drive in the social?

And if this were done by many or all of us who call ourselves *queer*, wouldn't it be some form of the associative, the common, the social? It would be a different matter if it were a form of irony – pardon the rhyme – which Edelman himself considers "the queerest of rhetorical devices", and which David Halperin, as I have already pointed out, locates as a strategy of subversion of genres: from the tragic to the comic, from the dramatic to comedy and vice versa. The heteronormative perspective is described as serious, categorical, sententious, moralising, psychologising, literal. Halperin gives as an example what happens when watching a comedy as "a documentary that tries to deal with serious psychological and social problems". For this view, the sentiments must not show their performative character; they must be far removed from any theatricality, they must be "authentic", and they cannot make any complicit or critical wink to the audience that would dismantle the device.

At this point, I must say that both Edelman and Halberstam seem to be more on the side of the *straight gaze*; they are extremely serious. And I will not miss this opportunity to add grist to my/our mill. Lacan now appears to me more of the *queer* side, for his humour, his irony, his *discursive dilettantism.* Don't worry, I'm sure we would have to relativise dilettantism, although some dictionary defines it as a liking for various arts or practices and not being a professional at something, which I don't think he would dislike too much.

Perhaps Edelman "rescues himself" – to use a prison jargon so much in vogue – gets funnier, when he creates the neologism *Sinthomosexuality*, in clear allusion to *Lacan's Synthome*, symptom, holyman, *santotomasdeaquino*, possible names for Joyce? In that Seminar, *Lacan* never ceases to surprise me – for better and for worse – all the time. For example, when he says that "as he had a rather loose willy, if I may say so, his art made up for his phallic firmness" or "his art is the true guarantor of his phallus", in short. . . . On the other hand, there are more than salutary hits – not in the sense of health but in the sense of health – such as: "the Name of the Father is also the Father of the Name", which would be enough for a lot of work if there were time.

Sinthomosexuality will then designate the particular way in which each subject succeeds in knotting the Real, Symbolic, and Imaginary registers. The homosexuality contained in the neologism would carry the weight of the non-sexual relation, would make its absence visible, and would make it possible to figure the availability of jouissance – Edelman maintains here the French term: *jouissance* – and, furthermore, the end of fantasy. Of course, it is not clear, at least to me, how this would come about.

As far as the end of fantasy is concerned, it would be interesting to question precisely fantasy and its traversal, something that Allouch also did in Buenos Aires.

Edelman is less clear to me when he says: "we sinthomosexuals . . .", because then it seems to me that some kind of community is already taking shape and my radical anti-everything enthusiasm of the beginning, with which I thought I was accompanying him, vanishes without return.

Finally, I return to Halberstam, who takes an unambiguous political stance. In a decidedly haranguing tone, he calls for

> creating a queer project that operates cooperatively with the other heads of the monstrous entity that opposes global capitalism . . . defining queer as a way of creating alternatives with others . . . an obscene, exaggerated and completely accessible queer negativity . . . etc.

I think I will again have to remain halfway in my expectations of the negative. Taking up Jacques Lacan's gauntlet when he is surprised to *still* be here, *not wanting to know about it*, and warning that we will have to sweat a lot, I will continue to sweat.

Of a power that is not exercised: Presentation in two acts[3]

How to begin

1 From where do we authorise ourselves to speak about something, someone, some people? This question haunts me every time I speak. Without pretending to be an unnecessary *coming-out*, which, moreover, I would never demand of

anyone, I nevertheless believe that – at least in psychoanalysis – there is an ethics of saying, which also includes writing, and presupposes at least a certain warning as to what we speak about and in what way. Jean Allouch prefers to speak of legitimacy. Perhaps that is more accurate, I don't know.

2 For almost ten years I was part of the team working with transsexuals in the Department of Medical Psychology at the Faculty of Medicine. There we received applicants for sex reassignment surgery and "followed them" for two years. Follow-up was the word used with a view to a diagnosis on which it would depend whether or not the person in question would agree to the requested operation. The *Diagnostic and Statistical Manual, fourth edition (DSM IV)*was the definitive psychopathological grid on which we were to base our recommendation, although, since most of us in the department called ourselves psychoanalysts, the report allowed for supposedly analytical considerations in a psychoanalysis-psychiatry pairing that we did not care for. However, on the occasion of my degree thesis ii: *Transsexuals: a possible approach*, and as a result of Lacanian approaches to the transsexual that is intended to be The woman with a capital letter, I wrote timidly:

> Or could it be that, for lack of any other signifier to name her, she is called a woman? Although I would say it differently today, I am happy to note that my subjection to this knowledge was at least not absolute, even at that time.

3 When I was younger, I believed that what mattered, what was important, was to say something original, unique, new, something that would be attached to my own name, enriching it, preventing it from falling. I didn't know what that meant! Of course, later analysis and life, my life and the lives of those I take into my supposedly analytical practice, have made me see how undesirable this idea is. The aim is not necessarily to "be spoken" by others – not necessarily in agreement or disagreement – but to pass on some of the ways of welcoming and rejecting what has come to be called queer theory.

Act 1: First voice

A Mexican psychoanalyst, whom I shall call El hombre in this commentary, which does not abjure a certain fictionalisation, gives a confession,[4] in which he raises the *need* to make a critique of gender theories from the perspective of psychoanalysis. In it he raises what I interpret as his alarm: a *zone of equivocation* among psychoanalysis, feminist theories, and cultural and social studies.

This Lacanian – remember that Lacan suggested being Freudian not Lacanian – denounces an alliance between constructivism – of which he makes *Foucault* one of its representatives – and the market and science on the basis of the postulate "your body is yours", which he ascribes to gender theories. He speaks of the eradication of the experience of the real by a nomadic subjectivity, of which it seems that *Foucault* is also guilty, of the elimination of structures, including the unconscious as a structure.

Says El hombre: "it is interesting that under the influence of Foucault there are even certain Lacanian psychoanalysts who question that there are structures". He speaks of a subject that rejects any subjection and finds in scientific advances its best ally, of identification to an ideal of equality – ideals are always totalitarian and hegemonic, he seems to say. The otherness of the body is unknown, he says. And he continues: an imaginary component dominates "your body is your body"; the body does not belong to us entirely, he reminds us. The self is not the master in its own house, the real dimension of jouissance is unknown as well as Extimacy (Lacanian neologism). Anatomy is destiny, a Napoleonic dictum taken up by Freud, which would have been a reference for Lacan when faced with a so-called psychotic patient with transsexual delirium. The real body does not cease to be an unavoidable mark, says this good Lacanian. He recalls the formulas of sexuation with the inscription on the masculine or feminine side: "every being who speaks is inscribed on one side or the other", and adds: "it will never be the same for a woman to inscribe herself on the masculine side as for a man, nor for a man to inscribe himself on the feminine side as for a woman, there will be some difference". – The man seems calmer after saying this.

It is interesting that the patient, said transsexual, said psychotic, in response to an intervention by Lacan: "You waited, you mean there was a hope", replies: a hope and an experience. An experience . . . isn't there also something of a real not to be ignored, I ask myself? But let's continue listening to El hombre: he takes up Foucault and refers to the relationship with boys; then, to the relationship with women – a subject that Jean Allouch recently, from a very different place, referred to in 2015 during his visit to Montevideo. The phantasmatic framework that frames jouissance is taken up again by El hombre in relation to female jouissance as a figure of excess and the Lacanian affirmation: "woman is a symptom of man", which seems to please him. "Woman is a symptom for those who are hindered by their phallus", he clarifies.

She alludes to Nora Joyce (Nora Barnacle) in Brenda Maddox's biography: "Nora is important because she belonged to Joyce and she has never belonged to him, the woman is always hetero". And he returns to the real of jouissance: "it is impossible not to enjoy", jouissance is above all autoerotic. The partner is not another. It is jouissance, he affirms. Then he visits the masochism of jouissance, the entry into the symbolic order, the loss of being and the fundamental fantasm, the symbolic identification and sexual identity. It eliminates – says El Hombre, alluding to gender theories – the subject's responsibility for his or her choice of jouissance. The "no sexual relation" implies a phantasmatic supplement, the encounter with the inconsistency of the Other (which The Man blithely assimilates to the parents).

And he continues: what does the Other want? is only answered with a new question, a new demand. The discourse of gender – this is how he locates it as a discourse, and once again Foucault is found guilty – sets out to invent itself in ignorance of all structure. And at the height of his alarm, he warns us: the unconscious would disappear! There is a remainder of jouissance that makes a symptom and everyone will have to make do with it, he concludes.

The curtain falls, everyone applauds, someone had to say all these things! Well, evidently The Man, like Manene, Lacan's sister, knows.

Act 2: Second voice

Quite another is the position, the way in which Jean Allouch – to name someone from the school of which I am a member – approaches these questions in a text that, among others, determined my act by which I expressed my desire to be a member of this school – of psychoanalysis – not of psychoanalysts.

Let us look at some of this text entitled *Avergonzados* (2005):

> On 23 November 2003, in Paris, the École Lacanienne de Psychanalyse (ELP) and the association Caritig (Centre d'Aide, de Recherche et d'Information sur la Transsexualité et l'Identité de Genre) organised a day for members of their respective communities, focusing on two related issues:
>
>> This was the first time in France, at least, that psychoanalysts and transgender people met in the same room and on the same platform. Until then, psychoanalysts talked about transsexuals (without having had any kind of encounter, they did not mind writing about them at all); this time: they talked to them.
>
> The debate was opened by the recent French translation of *Sex Changes (Le mouvement transgenre, changer de sexe*, Paris Epel, 2003), one of the many works of Pat Califia, first Patricia, then Pat and finally Patrick.
>
> There is a naming issue in this whole affair, which I think is not minor – although I can deal with it today – *Beatriz Preciado is now Paul Preciado, Judith Halberstam is now Jack Halberstam, Leonor Silvestri is now Leo Silvestri*. This is not the case with gay male activists and intellectuals, which would be interesting to think about.

Allouch continues:

> Now the Lacanians, however, widely summoned that day and being so open to the other – isn't it true? – distinguished themselves on the occasion by an abstention that had all the air of a *noli me tangere*.
>
> As far as I was concerned, the question was formulated as follows:
>
> Did I have the legitimacy to preside over one of the two sessions? This question came to me from a long time ago, in Argentina. In fact, while I was giving a seminar in Cordoba, one of the participants thought he could hand me a photocopy of *Sex Changes*. I concluded that I was considered susceptible, because of the words I had spoken, to receive this remarkable gift. This person was born

with a congenital malformation medically designated as Rokitanski Syndrome, with no vaginal cavity and no uterus, but with a vulva and distinctive secondary sexual characteristics. As a teenager, his father consulted Spanish doctors.

> The psychoanalysts, who in turn consulted the opinion of a psi, who, from the height of her knowledge, concluded: she was a girl, and so be it said. Only, lo and behold, *she knew herself to be a boy* – which was followed by a very painful and repeated surgery. Question:
>
> Is a psychoanalyst justified in decreeing someone's *gender*, in telling someone and their environment where they stand in the erotic?
>
> To play the expert? The answer is no, and that concerns each and everyone.
>
> A psychoanalysis does not identify in a genre, if it so identifies, it is not a psychoanalysis. In other words: the object of desire does not lend itself to being represented. This expert, I must point out now, was Lacanian. His taking sides commits each and every one of the members of the same community. It testifies to the fact that Lacanian psychoanalysis has not been able to hold its place (. . .)
>
> Hold its place? That means staying radically out of medicine and out of pastoral care . . . so that, at last, the Lacanian movement ceases to be insensitive to what is contemporary to it in erotics. Time will tell what part of illusion is behind such a gamble".

And in the same text, Allouch places castration on the side of castration:

> to have to endure breasts when you are a woman for a man, a penis when you are a man for a woman; it is to be imaginary emasculated. "Imaginary" doesn't mean that it doesn't count, does it?

He ends his text by recounting his meeting with Patrick Ythier, the French translator of *Sex Changes*, who is female-to-male (ftm) "just after the operation that freed him of his breasts and before a planned vaginoplasty" (I must thank Fer Monza for pointing out an error or slip-up here, which we do not know whether it is the author's or the translation's and which we will not be the ones to sanction otherwise: it should read hysterectomy not vaginoplasty, which is exactly the opposite).

> Then such radiant happiness leapt into my face . . . that I had no choice but to realise that I had never seen such a thing in any Lacanian psychoanalyst. I was then ashamed of myself, ashamed of Jacques-Marie Lacan, who, receiving a transsexual for his presentation of the sick, had words that I would not wish to reproduce, shame on myself for having so late taken the position I am speaking of here, shame on the Freudian movement. Everything happened as if Jacques-Marie Lacan had forgotten his ternary, and thanks to this forgetfulness, the old "reality" came out of his pocket, the same one that his ternary was refusing . . .

We have Freud's soul rejoiced and our theory confirmed. It's easy to put aside that, elsewhere, without us even knowing it, thank God, the price will be paid. . . . No, I didn't have the legitimacy to chair the first session of a colloquium bringing together trans and psychoanalysts, that was clear". To allow oneself to know what the mental health of another is, that is power. If psychoanalysis has an interest, a scope, an impact, in a word, a specificity, it can only be that of radically refraining from exercising that power on which psychiatry and psychopathology are founded. The psychoanalyst is given a power that he does not exercise, unless he abandons his function as a psychoanalyst.

(Allouch, 2005)[5]

Recently, working on texts by David Halperin, with Sandra Filippini and Diego Nin, we have been considering that there is, however, a dimension of power – in the Foucauldian sense – that is not exercised (in the strong sense of the term) and nevertheless operates in analysis.

How else could transference produce effects?

I won't say much more. Only that I understand that the queer field does not cease to raise questions. The psychic, identifications, masculinity and femininity, love, humour, suffering, the social bond, and the death drive are just some of the points open to crossover.

When Judith Butler (2015) interrogates the identification in the psyche-cultural norms relationship and says:

But what if these two dimensions cannot be dissociated from each other? Why distinguish between a suffering imposed on a person by violent, normalising cultural norms and a suffering that seems to emerge from within transgender identification? What makes us think that such identifications do not occur in relation to norms? And what makes us think that these norms do not operate precisely through the regulation or infiltration of identificatory practices?

And when Judith Halberstam (2008) proposes the expression *feminine masculinity* as a marker, an index, and a term to study creative ways of being queer people?

Or When Javier Saez (2015) says: *Love* is heterosexual:

I wonder if the rhetoric of love is just another discourse and another practice that we have adopted from the heterosexual regime. In any case, it is a totally harmless and domesticated discourse, something that does not bother the patriarchal and homophobic system at all. On the contrary, buns, queers and even trans people are much better digested and accepted when they have pareja ("what healthy boys, they are no longer promiscuous").

Or when David Halperin (2015) proposes gay-queer *humour* as a specific strategy for dealing with difficult and even dramatic situations such as AIDS:

> A mixture of glamour and abjection, a double register of an admiring imitation and a vengeful parody of a baroque and pathetic femininity, powerful, intense, perfect, at the same time extravagant and theatrical. Fragments of hetero culture which, taken out of context – and of gender, degenerated – acquire deviant, other meanings. It is not a matter of escaping the reality of pain, but of sharing it and thus confronting it, emptying the suffering of its pain, without denying it. By using one's own suffering in this way: as a vector of parody, one renounces sympathy, empathy, emotional consensus, emotional consensus, and the empathy, emotional consensus, identification, the mechanisms of social discredit are sabotaged".

Something of the social bond is at stake here in a different way.

Or again, Butler when she proposes to think of identification as discourse and as an address to someone in a context in which being recognised in language constitutes a part of the social reality in question. It is in the context of interpellation to an other with the request to be *named* differently.

Or Jack Halberstam (2015) and Lee Edelman (2014) or Bersani (1998) in their respective versions of a *queer negativity* or the *anti-social* in the gay. . . . It seems to me that none of this is alien to us and, I wish, I wish, as Fito Páez says: "we are up to the challenge".

Erotics of domination: Ranges of the act (presentation)[6]

Background

On this occasion, I was led to make a journey through what I felt called to do from a space that opened up under the signifier *Sur*, only provisionally. I knew it from the beginning . . . It was something to be dropped, but not before going through the edges of its occurrence, its necessary inconsistency but also its insistence . . .

Perhaps it was precisely its condition of being so "taken and brought", of being hackneyed, even of being manipulated, exceeded, emptied of meaning, that made it suitable for its signifying status . . . Perhaps.

That this movement had Mexico as one of its points of emergence – its position in the operation of invention of an America that claimed to be Latin is well known – was not indifferent to me.

That, on the other hand, art, and more precisely contemporary art, was given a place for the production of subjectivities and a paradigmatic quarry in which to receive and gather some of the Lacanian teaching could not fail to challenge me.

Something of the subjective constitution does not take place in the same way everywhere; something of the experience of bodies in relation to a land and a language, to a symbolic, an imaginary and a real that are not outside objective and subjective conditions of existence.

I could give some examples derived from my own experience.

I am not sure that this is the right place or the right moment. I will only say that only by attending to these particularities of the lived experience, to these "subtleties of the real" that had to do with a river . . . and a muddy, viscous bottom, through which it is necessary to pass on the journey towards the water . . . only by passing through it again was I able to get out of an impasse of a little over a year in my analysis. And that was not without someone in the position of an analyst making room for these marks, these traces, these inscriptions: *non-transferable.*

From the first colloquium in Mexico: *El Sur y sus sujetos desetes*, happily called "Seminario a voces", Duchamp's role was paired with that of *The Interpretation of Dreams*: "in the production of the definitive end of the Kantian subject", and with Lacan a further step was recognised in the notion of desire as desire of the Other, on the one hand, but also as desire caused by a very particular object: the object a.

Already there, the very operation of affirmative universal statements situated by Adorno and Horkheimer in their *Dialectic of Enlightenment* as part of the European Enlightenment was questioned. Postcolonial studies, among which Gayatri Spivac's (2003) text "Can the Subaltern Speak?" has an eminent place, were also necessarily – I am referring to a logical necessity. The very possibility of producing what is at stake. It was suggested that:

> a paradoxical effect can occur: the sub-versive productions of certain authors, for example Foucault or Deleuze, which in the French context have been corrosive for power, end up operating in the colonised countries as part of the dominant discourse through the cultural industry. (Argument of the *Seminar by voices. The South and its desiring subjects*).

How can we get out of the paradox whereby the destabilising authors of the culture of the North become in the South the status quo through which the colonising effect they claim to combat is generated? How can we generate the conditions to really speak when we live in the South? How to avoid making psychoanalysis an idealism?

Nor was I indifferent to the fact that it was in Sur, sur, sur, sur, sur . . . that Cuauhtémoc Medina, curator and now director of the University Museum of Contemporary Art (MUAC), posed for the field of art:

> Without denying the immense inequalities of power that define the operation of cultural production at the beginning of the century, what is certain is that the South has acquired a new critical and productive weight in the texture of the global imagination . . . a series of concentrations of energy are taking place that, by building complex networks, create institutions, markets and intellectual circuits that seek to differentiate themselves from the Euro-American operatives. Never before have artists from South America, Africa and Oceania had a similar opportunity for deployment. The South is not a region: it is a currency of invention, deviation and resistance.
>
> (2010)

Manuel Hernández (2013) in "La rotura y la vergüenza" speaks of "silencing effects". He says:

> Continuity and rupture (between subjugated culture and dominant culture) both occur through language, as Nahuatl is present in the Castellano spoken in the Valley of Mexico. Beyond a hybrid language that allows itself to be permeated by terms transposed from Nahuatl, such as *chocolate*, *avocado*, etc., there is a *mode of erotic relationship with the language that implies modes of subjectivation*, for example in the extensive use of diminutives, in the elaborate cut-and-paste of the Mexican that so astonishes foreigners, or in the sexuality played out in the albures. There is no subjectivity in the abstract . . ., what exists is a language that subjectifies in very specific erotic ways.

Erotics and language are presupposed. Coloniality as effects of colonialism, subjective, erotic, and linguistic effects. Subjective position, as an epistemic consequence of the Eurocentric claim to primacy in the production of meaning. Elimination of the tension of difference, of differences. Impossibility and powerlessness to pass on something of the language that constitutes us. Also as submission to the imaginary unity of the so-called Spanish language. Difficulty in making language work in its knowing-not knowing.

A southern position that was also for gay and lesbian studies and even more so for the vital experience of those of us who are named, alluded to, (dis)known, and whom it is not enough to welcome but it is still convenient to deploy, to bring to its limits, to enable consequences for psychoanalysis. Southern *Queer* Theory that will try to make those who do not feel said, said, said, said, said by the sex-gender system speak.

The queer in South America that with a Pedro Lemebel, a Nestor Perlongher, and a Reynaldo Arenas will say the queer in another way:

> "warrior queerness", "minority becomings", non-heteronormative becomings. Or, as Paola Arboleda Ríos (2011) points out in "ser o estar queer en latinoamérica . . .".

Despite the critical myopia of *queer* theories developed in Europe and North America, a significant number of artists, intellectuals, academics, gay and lesbian Latin American and US-born Latino authors (such as Gloria Anzaldúa and Cherríe Moraga) articulate their subjectivity and a good part of their intellectual proposal, not only in relation to their sexual dissidence but also in the face of multiple systems of oppression (class, race, ideology, etc.). Systems that intervene and are present in the construction of the socio-political reality of each of their countries and that have even led many of them to the so-called "sexilio" in search of power-being (Guzmán, 1997).

On one occasion when I was invited to participate in a meeting of the *Queer* Area, feminist members of Mundo Afro were invited, who with the forcefulness of those who have lived what they speak and for what they speak, said: "there is no feminism, but rather feminisms; for example, it was not a conquest for black women to go out to work, we always did that as employees or prostitutes". *Sur de sures de otros sures* to continue thinking.

Southern drifts: Textual performance

N'est pas sur

i.

. . . and when it seemed that there would be no more . . . that there would be no more . . . amidst vicissitudes and misunderstandings – may they never fail! not to elude, as Lacan would say to Dolto – in drifts that threaten misdirection and misencounters, and at the same time open up the possibility of misplaced encounters, in the oxymoronic dimension that is proper to us, the South also insists . . . and sorrow is followed by joy and illusion, and it is known that in this (un)chained succession we will alternate states, we will escape from dream to nightmare, from impotence to impossibility, from mistake to slip, again and again and again, and we will have to give up a lot so that something remains, at least something, and sustaining itself without consisting, insisting, resisting, and leaving its trace, some trace that we won't know if we produce it in act or if it produces us in the illusion of producing it, of producing the illusion of no future, the coming of no illusion and yet and yet . . . we will continue to sweat, to walk sud, *sur que n'est pas sur*, of course not, and still not wanting to know anything about it . . . when it seemed that no more, that no more . . .

. . . to bear witness to "the sorrow that has wounded me" and that even today, perhaps not for long, I decide to continue saying it south, renouncing some north, some norths, to try to give an account of the singular, very singular and not so singular way in which each one of us is marked, not only by a language but by some material and historical conditions and by other subjective and social conditions in the *distribution of the sensible.*

. . . and how these marks demarcate limits and possibilities of saying, of saying oneself without infinitely widening the field of an alienation that constitutes us – dismisses us once and for all, but not forever, but from time to time, so that something insubstantial and fleeting is said to be subject at the same time as it enables the fall of some rest, deject, abject object of desire.

. . . and this will not be possible unless we allow ourselves to be intervened, to be parasited, to be told, by a language that will not be Saussure's or Chomsky's, unless we make room for a knowing-not knowing of a language, our language, in the way the poet traces the echoes of something that speaks, speaks to him, makes him his scribe, his alienated and his secretary, in a madness that cures, cures him of being someone, being a desert and a jungle of words only apparently loose, uncluttered, fired, before any course, and with an enjoyment in the background, which can defund any saying.

ii.

. . . beautiful ideas seduce us they wiggle like a beautiful woman or a beautiful man there is nothing written about tastes my grandmother used to say and she was wrong there is too much written too much as of almost everything the writing saturates the subject the subjects and one no longer knows if it is text or meta-text although perhaps there are only meta-texts that follow one another infinitely in a relentless logic of production reproduction crisis of super-production. We will have to throw some of them or many of them or almost all of them almost everything into the river or the sea and start creating again to recreate the monster of reason the reasoning monster that is not *rocinant* I wish it were and would lead us far away to unravel entanglements that would become even more entangled and there will be no hand or monkey to undo it unravels and unburdens itself in an enjoyment the suffering enjoyment of love that is roma and mora sweet dwelling of the *ca* – the walking whaler saturated with static static still metastatic hypertexts that still the madwoman of the house who marries no one and with everyone she copulates and is annulled to the sweet sound of a ladi – no mean Latin hip hop that speaks of things that supposedly happen to seduce the man or the woman, both or neither of them?

iii.

. . . and like Pedro Lemebel, *mariquita linda*, el (la) del *barroco desclosetado*, as Carlos Monsivais (2007) said, to say: "I speak for my difference, or I am not Pasolini asking for explanations" (Lemebel, 1997). To speak because one has a broken wing, like everyone else, but something different, because the subalternities are added and one can be poor and black and whore and ugly or fat, and one can grow up hearing as an insult one's own traits, one's own-improper-appropriate ways, from the most traditional "*a que te den por culo*" – as if that were necessarily a disgrace – to the most South American chupaverga or *mamón* or *mamadera*, as if to say submissive or pimp, or hearing "*marica*" as weakness or fear, and in this short-circuit of meaning, opting to preserve the antithetical meaning of some words that tell us to un-tell us, making any speculative jubilation impossible and making that other is me, a me is another very other, too other of all otherness, only subjectivable from pain and humiliation.

. . . and we will have to be careful not to adopt pride inadvertently and welcome in the appropriation of a signifier the phallic glow that sustains it without being able to make it undergo a change of true sign or at least try to do so, and to do the same in reverse with its counterpart shame, not dismissing it by considering it only in its condition of stigma but doing something else with it in its relation to the real and the possibility of another crossing with the logos . . .

. . . Lemebel (2013) already knew this, and he says so in *CróniCas de nueva york. El Bar Stonewall:*

> What if one is invited to New York with all expenses paid to participate in the Stonewall event, twenty years after the police beating of the gay girls who in

1964 took over a bar in the Village neighbourhood. What if one is told the story and feels obliged to make the sign of the cross at the site of the event. A dark little bar, a shrine to the homosexual cause, where tourists come to lay their floral offerings.

Because there, in the showcase, are displayed the faded photos of the veteran hippie women who resisted the harassment of the law for I don't know how many days, the police aggression that tried to evict them without success. So how could one not shed a tear in this grotto of Lourdes Gay, which is like a sacred altar for the thousands of visitors who take off their Calvin Klein visors and respectfully pray for a few seconds when parade in front of the bowling alley. How can you not at least pretend to be sorry if you are a visitor in New York and you are being starved to death and paid for everything by these militant gringas who are so sanctimonious and commercial with their political history. How can you not politely pretend to be moved by those faces in the black and white photos, which could be from an old film we never saw, those photos of the gay heroes as if they were straight out of Woodstock, crowned with roses and coloured ribbons in the window of the Stonewall bar, the same as in the whole block, the same as in the whole Village, decorated like a pancake in the garb of the coloured fashions. Because when you get off the underground at Christopher Street you're suddenly confronted by a ton of muscle-heads and bodybuilders, in mini-shorts, bald and hooped, pairs of men on roller skates blowing past you as if they don't see you. And how are they going to see you if you are so ugly and dragging around the world your malnutrition of a third world madwoman. How are they going to look at you if you wear this astonished Chilean face in front of this olympus of powerful, well-fed homosexuals who look at you with disgust, as if to say: We're doing you the favour of bringing you, *indiecita*, to the cathedral of gay pride. And one is so absent-minded in these scenes of the Big World, looking at the shops full of sadomasochistic fetishes, nails, safety pins and screws and pins and all kinds of metal crap to torture one's skin. Oh what a pain! How frightening to see on the corner that group of Leaders with their motorbikes, moustaches, leathers, boots and that fascist brutality that reminds you of the macho gangs that in Chile you used to do the same to them, cross the street and walk stiffly, looking the other way. But here in the Village, in the little square in front of the Stonewall bar, there is plenty of that male power that makes you panic, that dwarfs you like a little Latin fly standing in this neighbourhood of blonde sex. In this sector of Manhattan, the pink zone of New York where things are worth an arm and a leg, the epicentre of the commercial tour for homosexuals with dollars visiting the city. Especially on this global holiday when the island of Manhattan is decked out in all the colours of the gay rainbow. Which is more like just one, white. Because maybe gay is white . . .".

. . . a Lemebel, a pretty Chilean South American sissy, who will change his name to Beatriz Preciado, Paul from now on, as an intimate homage to the one for whom it was obvious that she, that is to say he, was called Paul and not Beatriz, and whom he will mourn with rage and gratitude on his death:

> Fucking AIDS, fucking cancer of the larynx, fucking dictatorship and fucking democracy, fucking macho mafia that they still call a party, fucking censorship, fucking couples and fucking break-ups, fucking Pedro and fucking Paco, fucking television, fucking alternative movements, fucking socialism, fucking colonial church, fucking NGOs, fucking pharmaceutical multinationals, fucking post-dictatorship neoliberal farra, fucking map of the Southern Cone, fucking cultural consensus, fucking tourism, fucking tolerance, fucking art biennials and fucking museum of homosexuality. Fucking you and fucking me. Fucking your body that has lost. And fucking your soul that will never lose. Fucking the minority crowd in front of a single armed man. Whores the mares and whores the Mapocho River. Whores the days we spent together in Santiago, whores the nights in Valparaíso, whores your kisses and whores your tongue. We looked at the Pacific and I quoted Deleuze: "The sea is like cinema, a moving image". You said to me: "Don't be an intellectual, macho man. The only moving image is love". You brought me up and from you I came out as a son, one of the hundreds you had, invented by your voice. You are my mother and I cry for you as one cries for a transvestite mother. With a dose of testosterone and a *grito*. You are my mother and I mourn you as one mourns a communist and indigenous mother. With a hammer and sickle drawn on the skin of my face. You are my shaman mother and I cry for you as one cries for ayahuas- ca.
>
> (Preciado)

. . . and then in the superficiality and the sinking and reappearing and reigning no kingdom, between other skins, other skins, dripping the felony of life, dripping erratic, erratic, erratiques, erratic, in the proximity of miracles that will not happen, we will perhaps retrace something of a path traced by others with lower case letters but not so similar and with capital pretensions.

. . . the south also insists.

Importunate psychoanalysis: Importuning and being importuned

Since its birth and for a long time, psychoanalysis has been bothering the consciences of the West, and at the same time – this will be my hypothesis today – it is the effect of something that is bothering.

If *importunar*, according to the Real Academia Española, is "to *incomodar* or bother with an insistent or inopportune claim or request", we should ask ourselves: what was that claim or request of psychoanalysis? And if, furthermore, etymologically, to importune is to impede the passage of something, what would it have been about? I will not hasten to answer.

In 1968, in the first session of the seminar *From an Other to the Other*, Lacan (2008a) declares himself to be bothered by Marx. He does not say concerned, involved, touched . . . he says importuned, that is to say, annoyed, solicited, intervened by. Lacan will allow himself to be intervened, pestered, without this resulting in any kind of ideological subjugation, but not without consequences for him and his field of practice: psychoanalysis.

The result of a traffic between dissimilar fields of knowledge, using homology as an operation and complex language passages, the plus valence will make room for the *plus de jouir*. From this will derive effects for analytic practice: "I will turn to Marx, whose words, troubled as I have been for a long time, I regret not having introduced earlier into a field where he is nevertheless perfectly in place" (Lacan, 2008a).

It is not at all obvious that it can be done that way; the ways of doing or doing with . . . are fundamental. I don't know how else to put it in a way that convinces me of what feminisms, *queer* theory, and decolonialism are importing to psychoanalysis today. What is certain is that we cannot ignore it or deny it by saying: "that's not psychoanalysis." Not anymore!

But what are the things with which psychoanalysis is bothered? The answer is so simple as to be absurd: everything. And surely some Lacanian will remind me of Lacan's not everything, *pas tout*, and so I will sharpen my aim: psychoanalysis finds itself impeded in its not-everything. Not because it is necessary to return to some kind of totality – quite the contrary – but because perhaps it is time to review how not-all this not-all is, if it excludes exclusions that constitute and institute it.

I pass in review: psychoanalysis has been troubled[7] by the notions of man, woman, Oedipus, phallus, castration, sexual difference, active-passive, love . . . Is it necessary to continue? I add the questions insisted upon by decolonial theories or intersectionality: is psychoanalysis a Eurocentric invention from a colonial logos? is there room for something else? what can psychoanalysis say about the racialisation of bodies or poverty and class? what can it say, not only about its subjective effects but also about the very production of the subjective there?

More recently, since the so-called *affective turn* in the queer field, affects seem to have begun their disaggregation from what David Halperin (2015) in *How to be Gay* calls "the heterosexual dramaturgy of affects". Already in that text, Halperin warned about the heterosexual matrix that runs through the consideration of the affective, taken as universal. A heterosexual matrix that makes affects a place of subjective truth, denying them any performative and political character. For this matrix, there would be only one way of experiencing what we call mourning, sadness, joy, pain, etc. *Queer* experience disproves this supposed universality or affective normativity.

The multiple, parodic, performative ways in which the gay community confronted the AIDS pandemic are just one demonstration of this, so there is no longer a single way of dealing with it. As Laurent Berlant, Nicolás Cuello, Mariela Solana, Ann Cvetkovich, Sara Ahmed, and many others have pointed out – from differential biases in each case – there is a political dimension of affects, or as I prefer to say: a *political economy of affects*. Affects affect, do something, perform. So it is no longer possible to situate them as the site of a truth of the subject.

Paul B. Preciado (2019b), on the occasion of his intervention at the 49th Conference of the École de la Cause Freudienne: *Women in Psychoanalysis*, has come to disturb us:

> the regime of sexual difference that you know and consider as universal and quasi-metaphysical, on which all psychoanalytic theories are based and articulated, is neither an empirical reality nor a founding symbolic order of the unconscious. It is nothing more than an epistemology of the living, an anatomical cartography, a political economy of the body and a collective management of this reproductive energy.
>
> It is a historical epistemology that is constructed in relation to a racial taxonomy, as much as to European mercantile and colonial development, and which crystallises in the second half of the nineteenth century.
>
> This epistemology, far from being the representation of a reality, is a performative machine that produces and legitimises a specific political and economic order: hetero-colonial patriarchy.

Preciado adds:

> It is interesting to think that Freudian psychoanalysis, as a theory of the psychic apparatus, as a clinical practice, appears precisely at the moment when the central notions of the epistemology of sexual difference are crystallised: man and woman defined as anatomically different and complementary in their reproductive potency, as potentially paternal and maternal figures, respectively, in the colonial, bourgeois family institution; but also heterosexuality and homosexuality thought of as normal and pathological, respectively.
>
> Psychoanalysis, seen from the angle of the history of the abject body, the history of the monster of normative sexuality, and the science of the unconscious, patriarchal and colonial.

Preciado proposes, by importuning us, to situate psychoanalysis in a *genealogy of the abject body*.

In the beginning, it was the women who bothered the Medina and Sigmund Freud. In the beginning, it was the body of the so-called hysterics that stood in the way and prevented the continuation of the medical discourse. Freud was good enough to keep quiet and listen. He gave up his privileged position to crazy, crazed women, who made themselves heard through their speaking bodies. Later, it would be another woman, Margueritte, or Aimé, who would disturb Jacques Lacan, this time from another mode of madness. And psychoanalysis will once again be the *invention of madness*, as Jean Allouch (2020) rightly points out:

> Psychoanalysis was and remains an invention of madness. This feature distinguishes it from related disciplines (psychiatry, psychology, psychopathology,

criminology) which all come from society and serve it. Their formula is: "Society must be defended". Thus crime was regularly seen as an attack on life in society, and murderers were condemned for it, from the very beginning of the reports of psychiatric and judicial bodies. Psychoanalysis dug its fragile place . . . elsewhere, next to those whom society rejects. I call it a "pariasitarian" discipline. It is not on the side of those who have the upper hand, where people are told how to think and, above all, how to behave.

You need to have dealt closely with madness, to have stumbled upon it with the clairvoyant eyes of a child in order to one day, later on, have wanted to practice psychoanalysis – which is still madness.

Perhaps something of this being bothered makes *being an analyst* in psychoanalysis. Something of this availability to what makes an obstacle, to what pushes-pushes to be heard-read is a trait not to be dropped, if we still want to call ourselves psychoanalysts. Of course, as long as we know that we are not psychoanalysts except in the analytic act, and even there we are not psychoanalysts all the time.[8] That is why I propose that perhaps it would be better, more in line with what happens in an analysis, to say that *we are analysts*. We are analysts when we make appearance; but semblance is a technical term of Lacan of the objects that are the cause of the analysand's desire in analysis. The rest of the time, in the best of cases, we are in the position of analysands, supposing subjects to a knowledge and knowledges to a subject.

But this makes us uncomfortable, and it is not uncommon for us to see our position as that of master. Then a university discourse passes itself off as an analytic discourse, and we think we have thus eliminated the discomfort that never ceases to bother us.

If it is in the position of analysands that something of *a knowledge that does not know itself* can pass into our saying psychoanalysis, it will only be from an uncomfortably singular implication that we speak.[9] Enunciative position and the practice of saying – if we are talking about psychoanalysis – can no longer be dissociated.

Of course, we know from Foucault, and also from Lacan, that the personal is political – albeit from a different slant – that saying is not outside discourse. In Foucault, discourse will be part of the dispositif, while in Lacan it will be the dispositif itself. We move from an uncomfortable position between that which we believe to be singular and that for which we are spoken-said. There is also an unresolved tension between a saying, which is always a saying of the jouissance that causes us, and a not wanting to know anything about that jouissance. We psychoanalysts are the ones who resist psychoanalysis, what is unbearable in it, but at least we are aware of it . . .

Discourses will then be devices of articulation, of localisation of that jouissance that imports all discourse. Leo Bersani (2011) shows this very well in his book *The Freudian Body*. According to the author, there was something deeply disturbing in Freudian findings, even for Freud himself, which caused him to divide into two currents or biases: one more speculative and the other more theoretical. The speculative bias sought or made it possible to remain very attached to the disclosures, while from the theoretical point of view, "domesticating clarities of narrative orders" were established.

How can we live up to that which is importuning us? Or at least, how can we not play the sad role of erasing with our elbow what we write with our hand? As Thamy Ayouch (2020) reminded us not so long ago, psychoanalysis is a practice of hybridity:

> Through its epistemological mixtures, psychoanalysis seems to provoke a denaturalisation of the models it borrows: those are no longer specific to a particular epistemology, but become modelizations, susceptible of interweaving to designate a process of enunciation.

Perhaps it is precisely to the particularity of this hybridisation that we can call psychoanalysis. Hybridisation of discourses: medical, literary-mythological, philosophical, and of knowledge: of bodies, of speech, of minor, rejected, repressed, oppressed knowledge. Multiple operations, traffics, language passages, invention . . . this is what it is all about in this reception of the contemporaneity of what troubles us.

As I have already pointed out, I am part of a school that long ago embraced *gay and lesbian studies* and queer theory, as well as Foucault, Deleuze, and Guattari, a political act or gesture from the analytical field, not without consequences. These will operate towards the rest of the so-called analytical community or Freudian field – it remains to be seen which community we are talking about, which field, as well as consequences and effects within the school. A school which, moreover, has made and continues to work on a difficult but sustained attempt to depathologise and demedicalise analytic practice.

We have already seen something of this gesture in *De un poder que no se ejerce*,[10] where Jean Allouch (2005), in his text *Avergonzados*, tells us how he experiences shame – that of Jacques Lacan, his own, and that of all of us, in the episode in which:

> Jacques-Marie Lacan, who, receiving a transsexual for his presentation of the sick, had words that I would not wish to reproduce, shame of myself for having taken so late the position I am speaking of here, shame of the Freudian movement. Everything happened as if Jacques-Marie Lacan had forgotten his ternary, and thanks to this forgetfulness, the old "reality" came out of his pocket, the same one that his ternary was refusing . . .

Could shame then be another of the names of *this importunium*? One that does not cease, for if anything can be called ethics, it will try to realise, to push to the limit, not to give in, to deploy this gesture in all its consequences so that it becomes an act.

Jean Genet ([1949] 1976) says in *Diary of a Thief* that acts are infamous for not being finished: "Acts must be pursued to their end. Whatever their starting point, the end will be beautiful. It is because it is not finished that an action is infamous". Let us then pursue this act that allows us to escape from that *psi function* that makes psychoanalysis a discipline at the service of the device of sexuality. And if I say discipline, believe me it is not innocent. Let us continue this act that makes it possible to make psychoanalysis an *erotology of passage* (Allouch, 1998) in which a logos does not annul an eros, in which from this impossible hybridisation a different practice is born each time, one that continues to disturb the spirits.

Not so long ago in another forum, I said that in this sense, something is beginning to open up, from the emphasis that Allouch (2017) has been placing for some time now on Lacan's "there is no sexual relation". Something that, in my opinion, would make it possible to leave behind the notion of castration and, probably, of lack. The inexistence of sexual relation, in the mathematical sense of writing, radicalises the logical impossibility of heterosexuality hitherto seen as obligatory or destiny. However, it is not obvious to me that it means dropping sexual difference, resulting from the sex-gender binarism as a system. Unless we conclude that there is no sexual relation *because there is no sexual*. Unless we stop regulating ourselves by difference and do so by the diverse and multiple.

Non-existence of the sexual relation that is also in the same act *non-existence of the sexual*, not to be *conquered* (I don't like any conquest) – I'm more seduced by saying: to be *realised* (playing with the real and the realisation)".

I know, I know, that it is a lot, perhaps too much of a gamble. I know that it probably borders on the impossible. But, if it is psychoanalysis, what else could be expected?

What heterosexuality owes to psychoanalysis

"Talking-hurt is a useful poetic and epistemic regime", says my Portuguese friend Daniel Lourenco. Let's give it a try. But before we begin, I think it is pertinent to make a clarification that has as its starting point an uninterrupted conversation that we have been having with the psychoanalyst and friend Sandra Filippini for some years now. I will refer to Uruguayan psychoanalysts without this being an *I accuse*, but rather to take their writings as analysers of a traversal.

Lacan says that it was Marx who gave discourse to capitalism, doing something different with the *obscure function* of surplus value. In this way, the invention of surplus value and the surplus of enjoyment are placed in homology; and it will be Lacan who will give discourse to psychoanalysis.

> Labour was not new in the production of the commodity, just as the renunciation of jouissance was not new . . . this renunciation constitutes the master. . . . The novelty is that there is a discourse that articulates this renunciation and makes what I will call the function of the surplus of jouissance appear.
>
> (Lacan, 2008b)

This operation is placed as the essence of analytic discourse

Giving discourse participates in the ambiguous possibility of making another discourse exist and produce another discourse, a possible way out of the real effects that each discourse produces. Of course, I am not saying that analytic discourse, in the sense in which Jacques Lacan understands and formalises it, is heterosexual discourse, but rather that it is psychoanalysis as university discourse, via science; it will be from there that a certain psychoanalysis will do its favours to heterosexuality. Nor do I speak of heterosexuality as eroticism and sexual practice – one among many – but as a political regime, in the sense given to it by Monique Wittig ([1992] 2006).

I therefore hypothesise that psychoanalysis, together with other disciplines, gave discourse to heterosexuality. In this sense, the location in the disciplinary is a provocation, I believe, not at all gratuitous. I am referring to medicine, and in particular to psychiatry, in the joint enterprise of biopower and the psi function that Foucault envisaged.

I open the umbrella: my reading will be biased, self-interested, neither objective nor neutral, neither exhaustive nor scientifically objectionable, fragmentary, and so on and so forth. But this is not a lack of method: this will be the method.

I will speak little or nothing of Lacan, of Foucault, and yet I will refer to what for some time now – from a rereading of the book *The Sinthome* (Lacan, 2006c) – has obsessed me: what Lacan calls there *practices of saying*. Because I believe that this is what it is all about, although this should not be understood as meaning that everything that happens in an analysis, much less outside of it, is about saying; unless we give saying an expanded field that includes various modes of doing: with and without words, silence, and so on and so forth.

Sample buttons . . . or how are we doing at home?

i.

Aida Aurora Fernández, in "Confusion and acting out. Some aspects of the analysis of a homosexual patient", a work that can be read online and that the Asociación psicoanalítica del Uruguay (APU) uploads with the following descriptors: male homosexuality/hypochondria/confusion/clivaje/acting out/primary defence/schizophrenia/schizophrenia mechanisms/hypochondriasis/confusion/clivage/acting out/primary defence/schizoid mechanisms/envy/voracity/integration/persecutory guilt/destruction/clinical case. To begin with, I think about what someone outside psychoanalysis would think if they were guided by these descriptors, and even more, I think about what these descriptors say about what we have naturalised, what has become jargon.

> In the first interview with Pablo, 25 years old, I am struck by his anxious and worried appearance. He came to me looking for a solution to his conflicts, sent by a psychologist, after having tried different psychiatric treatments. Immediately a warm communication was established between the two of us, *and although his*

history showed that homo-sexual practices had begun in his childhood, I sensed something in him that confirmed a nascent feeling that he might be recoverable.
(Italics are mine)

Later, in another session:

Next Wednesday's session. – Do you know what? I've been thinking that only here can I find the solution to all my doubts, to this dizziness that I feel inside me, not like an ordinary dizziness, but like walking around, talking, doing things and feeling that there are two of me, that one does what the other doesn't want to do? It's a hell of doubts inside me. I doubt everything . . . look, and I don't know anything, everything confuses me, help me, tell me what's wrong with me? What is it that's wrong with me?

I interpret: The doubts, the confusion, you feel them here with me, as *you don't know what I am, what I am like, if I am a woman, if I am a man, how you felt your parents confused as a child, who was the woman, who was the man. You don't know when you are here with me if you are a man, if you are a woman.*

Pablo: But I want to be me, myself, no matter what, whether something big or small, I don't care how, but to know what I am, how I am, I don't care about anything, as long as I am, I want to be me. It's like taking your head out of the water, drowning, and putting it back in and continuing to drown and not drowning, it's as if something is taking me away . . . I don't know what . . .

I interpret: He feels that he suffocates if he relates to me with his male part, he feels that he suffocates if he relates to his female part. He asks me to tell him what I am like, to know what you are; for me to define you, to tell him what he has to do with me.

"My mother used to tell me," Pablo continues, "no women, if you come home before 9 o'clock at night, and when I was a boy she wouldn't let me go around the block. to walk around the block. I'd go to the corner and shiver, I'd play with Tom, you know . . . (sexual games).

I interpret: Here I let him walk around the block, that's why he gets confused, he gets scared,

he does not know whether I am a woman, whether I am like Tom; he trembles because he does not know what you are like, when you are with me, whether half a woman as he feels his father or half a man as he feels his mother.
(Italics are mine)

And so the session continues. Later, he interprets:

He can't place me, just as he couldn't place his mother, his father, he *lived them confused, in their roles. The sick mother, but strong, authoritarian. The father a servant, weak with an apron (feminine parts).* The characteristic of confusion thus appears: a mixture of indiscriminate parts of a feminine

> object-sick-semi-destroyed, but authoritarian with phallic aspects (cuchillo-penis), and a masculine object-impotent-delivered.
>
> (Italics are mine)

In another session:

> Undoubtedly, in one aspect, it also has the character of a negation, insofar as *the masculine homosexual, in his delirium, denies the real existence of a man's body, in order to identify himself with his internal, de- seated-hated object (the mother-breast), a woman's body.*
>
> (Italics are mine)

The *homosexual* makes his appearance, substantivised, exemplary, universal. Practices of nomination, classificatory naming not without real effects. Or to quote Otto Fenichel: "The factor that primarily disturbs *genital primacy* is identical to that which produces the same effect in neurotics, anguish and feelings of guilt, directed against the Oedipus complex" (in Fernández, 1970), although he clarifies that with different results, due to the mechanisms at play. Genital primacy is disturbed; there is no possible problematisation of its primacy-supremacy.

ii.

Another Uruguayan analyst, Alberto Pereda (1968), in an article whose section he calls "Projection of the death instinct", states with regard to a homosexual patient:

> *The homosexual feels full of destruction and death, as a function of the excessively hostile relations with his destructive and persecutory inner objects and the terrifying fantasies that sustain them. Situations of frustration increase the intensity of his destructive experiences, he feels incapable of handling them alone, that death is all-pervasive and he fears the annihilation of his ego.* Homosexual acting-out allows him to alleviate his persecutory anxiety by projecting the death instinct onto his ego, "partenaire". The basic unconscious fantasy is that death is 'passed on' to the other".
>
> (Italics are mine)

It is then another evidence: there are internal objects that are distrusted and persecutory in a horror movie interior, the bad kind, of course. And this produces annihilation or its annihilating projection onto another. The death drive – here called instinct, in case we need to reinforce its innateness – does its work. And the analyst – I write it with a capital letter, parodying his existence, his consistency, his entification – will do his work of rescuing and protecting his patient and, why not, the threatened society.

iii.

Another analyst, Juan Vives (2014), addresses the issue of the practice of psychoanalysis by homosexuals in "Can homosexuals practice psychoanalysis?" I think his witty paraphrase of *Can lay people practice analysis* (Freud, 1988a) shows a relationship to medical knowledge-power that is not unrelated to this debate. He begins his article by stating: "Traditionally, people with some kind of sexual perversion – including homosexuality – have been barred from entering psychoanalytic institutes". What surprises us is the explicitness of something that for many was a rumour not easily verifiable. And one wonders:

> What would be the reasons why a homosexual subject should be rejected from psychoanalytic training, is homosexuality really a formal limitation for the practice of psychoanalysis, what is the basis on which a perversion – in this case homosexuality – should be excluded from the practice of psychoanalysis, what is the basis on which a perversion – in this case homosexuality – should be excluded from the practice of psychoanalysis?

Perversion is an evidence. And he continues his analysis:

> *Is homosexuality compatible with a "normal personality"; is there such a thing as a healthy homosexual? Is "homosexual identity" a deviant or a normal form of development?* In relation to arguments that a heterosexual orientation in object choice is the "normal" way, while a homosexual choice is "abnormal", the criteria that have been put forward over the last 150 years have been arguments anchored in the postulates of evolutionism. Homosexual couples – both male and female – are, by definition and by biological impossibility, sterile; therefore, they are subjects that do not enter into the game of survival of the fittest because they cannot pass on their genetic characteristics.

Deviance, development, healthy, but also survival, evolution, Darwinism . . . At least someone says the prurient things without shame, although perhaps from the violence of a descriptive innocence that is not beyond his position of privilege. And he continues to make institutional impudence public:

> On the other hand, political pressures and, why not say it, a certain veiled threat of recourse to the courts, have led to a declaration of non-discrimination, signed by the president of the ipa, in order to explicitly include the term homosexuality alongside those of race, creed, gender and skin colour.

Threats, courts, political pressure, declarations . . . The state, like a just father, will settle matters and say what is best for everyone. Vives denounces, in addition to the pressure political, the misrepresentation *of Freud* for political purposes:

> Freud's sentence of "they are not sick" must be contextualised in the sense of "they are not neurotic", given that it is a perverse expression of infantile sexuality – hence his insistence, in the same texts to speak of a "perverse orientation".

The reference to prayer, instead of Freud's "saying" or "the sentence", made me think of prayer as prayer, supplication, or plea. But that is surely a perverse deviation on my part. The author argues primarily with Roughton (2001a) and his work "Homosexuality: clinical and technical issues":

> this author . . . speaks of "societies [psychoanalytic] in which homosexuality is still considered a perversion and discrimination is still a fact", a statement that does not sift through or discuss the criteria for stating whether homosexuality is not or is not a perversion, It also fails to distinguish the fact that a nosological criterion does not constitute any justification for any kind of discrimination – which does not invalidate the use of guidelines based on the capabilities or limitations that a person (whether homosexual or heterosexual) may have for the performance of a function.

It adds:

> Not giving an airline pilot's licence to an epileptic does not imply discrimination, but a formal limitation inherent to his or her seizure disorder for the exercise of a profession. In the same way, when a diabetic child is restricted from eating sugary sweets or a haemophiliac child is advised not to join the boxing team, it would be difficult to claim that they are being discriminated against; on the contrary, in these cases, limiting means a form of protection.

At this point one wonders whether Jean Allouch's statement that "psychoanalysis will be Foucauldian or it will not be" will not already have an answer: it will not be.

My mother, in a sort of Nietzschean fervour, used to say to me: "you will be what you must be or you will be nothing"; and I liked to reply: "I will be nothing"; I ask you to excuse my association in all its ambiguity and ambivalence.

iv.

Finally, another analyst recently expressed his fear of subjective devastation by the fall of what he called "ternarial definitions" and which I will not resign myself to not renaming: holy trinities.

> Dufour also points out that this decline in ternary definitions has devastating effects on subjectivity. The primacy of a market that ignores the Third would, in this author's opinion, promote the indistinction of the sexes. There would be a link between the demands for the right to sexual choice and the triumph of

> the market. It would neither be a question of killing the symbolic Father, nor of defending the Patriarchy. Between negation and dogma, the challenge is to explore the new psychic "economies".

The author also echoes the warning of another analyst, Daniel Gil:

> The terrible figure of the imaginary father would reappear in the imperative to jouissance, with the exaltation of the diverse that characterises this epoch of liberation of the forms of eroticism and in which the place of the third party, of the law, appears to be questioned.

On the side of the so-called Lacanians, there are no fewer examples. Some of this I tried to show in "Of a power that is not exercised: presentation in two acts" (in this book).

Mea vergüenza

As my friend Sandra Filippini always reminds me, it is easier to see what is wrong, what is open to criticism, in others. So I *am ashamed* to say that in my first attempts to say something about an analytic practice, my own, begun very early on, I also showed the *thread* of the crossing of the heterosexual in psychoanalysis. In a paper I called "Being and seeming. Sexual identity and narcissism" (Barrios, 1993), I said about a case: "the sense of this work is a first attempt to analyse the complex relationship between the process of identity formation and the achievement of an adult sexual identity and its disorders".

For me to be horrified by it today would be no more than a guilty reaction. Something else, or something less, would have to happen to place this horror on the side of shame. The truth is that I was not alone in this wager; I was accompanied by authors of reference: Otto Kernberg, Herbert Rosenfeld, Heinz Kohut, and others. I will only say in a weak plea in my favour that the central bias of the work was more on the side of narcissism and the self than on the side of the "sexual identity", which today I put in quotations; however, it was not yet possible for me to question the very notions of identity and sexuality that at that time were compared from the hetero-normality standard.

Survival strategies? Today I consider that, in spite of this, I believed in the possibility of fissuring at some point that matrix, on the side of being, of the subjective constitution in a sort of "pre-sexual", "pre-genital" field. Today, my shame also passes through the exhibition of a case, which gives an account of what is unportable for me, while constituting an unnoticed intervention in it.

I feel that this work could have been called "On hetero-sexuality as destiny". I still remember the impact on me of these texts by Aída Fernández: "La belleza, fuente de terror y plenitud; enfoque psicoanalítico del conflicto entre el sentmiento ético y el estético" (1970), and another in which she spoke of the "perversion of the ethical by the aesthetic", in allusion to Oscar Wilde but generalised to homosexual artists at least. The beautiful prevailing (!) Common fate or neighbour of women with fragile superego? Today I can joke and take those absurdities for their absurd, coarse side . . . It was not always like that.

D. Halperin (2000) says in the Preface to the French edition of *Saint Foucault:* "Saint Foucault is a book animated by anger". At this point, it is not a minor fact that someone who is going through the age admits anger and pain in the production of writing. It is not minor in that it empowers others.

In times of assimilationist triumphalism, it is perhaps a good idea not to hide memories and experiences that have marked the analyses and lives of many. Let me lighten the matter with humour, without turning this into a heterodrama.

It is also in this text by Halperin that, in discussion with the philosopher Richard Mohr and his book *Gay Ideas*, the author recalls that Foucault also participated in this project of writing the history of sexuality "from the point of view of a history of discourses".

A possible genealogy of degenerate psychoanalysis[11] in me: Seven steps of a testimony

I have heard – and I like to believe it – that the only Seminar that Lacan regretted having given was called *The Ethics of Psychoanalysis*. Probably because of the inevitability of a moral drift, despite all the possible distinctions between ethics and morality. And because it would be a prescription, in addition to the idea that analysis is something more than that which is produced every time.

There is no ethics of psychoanalysis, it is said. However, I, more modestly, say that there is an ethics of writing in psychoanalysis – writing that is not at all obvious. If there is an ethic of writing in psychoanalysis, it is that of writing only about what concerns us, involves us, constitutes us. It is not a question of prescribing the *coming out*, which would be a contradiction in terms, but of wanting a certain warning that it is only possible to speak *from within ourselves*, that is to say, from this fabulation of identity, this somatopolitical fiction that we are and that we perform.[12] And incidentally, its counterpart, not to speak of others, about others, for others . . .

There is no ethics of psychoanalysis but there has been a norm: heteronormativity, oedipal heteronormality. However, something must have insisted for us to be here today "*demantelando*" – as Preciado says – if *mantellum* in Latin is also veil, unveiling psychoanalysis. Unveiling us.

i.

Many years ago, when I had to write my thesis for my second degree in medical psychology at the medical school in my country, I reluctantly left my doubts about sexual binarism there, at the request of my thesis tutor. Or when I wonder what Catherine Millot and other Lacanians mean when they say that *the* transsexual wants to be The woman with a capital letter.

ii.

Likewise, the first psychoanalytical work I presented and after years of working in the team receiving requests for gender reassignment surgery, I was faced with the question of what to say about it. What and how, which is also what?

Transsexuals in medical practice. A possible approach, that was the name of the thesis (I note that today I still insist on this formula that alludes to the possible and that the possible is always a possibility, not the only one: the title of this paper gives it away: A possible genealogy). Today I see what is left of that thesis in my possession: only articles submitted to journals. I must say that the copy of the thesis that remained in my hands disappeared. Did I lose it? Did I hide it from myself? Who knows . . .[13] I see that thesis as suffering stammerings, formations of compromise, words between the lines, between confusion, and the *semblance* of academic rigour.

Nevertheless, something seems to be said there that I could say better or at least with less anguish, starting with the confusion that the biblical sentence always generated in me: God created man in his image and likeness, male and female he created them, which made me think about what was then God's sex-gender, male and female, a non-binary God who established or pretended to establish an impossible binarism? The fatality of a binarism that constitutes what I would later understand as the *sexual politics of language*.

I published a round-up of these issues, albeit in a different way: *Being and Appearing. Sexual identity and narcissism*. It is a clinical case; I was not yet authorised to talk about the analysands, despite the measures, which today I see as naïve, to protect identity by changing the name and some biographical data.

In that text I said: "The sense of this work is a first attempt to analyse the complex relationship between the process of identity formation and the achievement of an adult sexual identity and its disorders"; and although today, with Monday's paper, almost everything written there should be reformulated: identity, sexual identity, adult, etc., at least I wish to rescue the reception of the complete, the timid attempt to denaturalise the sex-gender system operating in psychoanalysis and being operated by it. On the other hand, I allude – without knowing it, but knowing it – to the performative dimension of all identity.

I am not trying to say that I always knew that *psychoanalysis would either be degenerate or it would not be* – I am never entirely convinced by these formulas – I even believed that it was more a question of something that did not fit me than of a failure of psychoanalysis. It would take twenty-one years on the couch, twice or even three times a week, and as many years of practising psychoanalysis, before any of this could be said. And Lacan and Foucault, and Deleuze and Guattari, and Monique Wittig and Gayle Rubin, and Judith Butler and Preciado, and *gay and lesbian studies* and *queer theory*, and feminisms and decolonial theories, and contemporary art and literature, which would cross me and affect me in a thousand and one ways known and unknown to me until I can say, not without irony: there is life outside the sex-gender system and the dispositif of sexuality!

iii.

Not long ago, I presented a paper at a conference of the École Lacanienne de Psychanalyse in Montevideo, which I provocatively called: "What heterosexuality owes to psychoanalysis". I believe that psychoanalysis contributed something not minor to heterosexuality – understood as a political regime, in Monique Wittig's sense – some psychoanalysis, yes, but in this case one could say "Psychoanalysis", since Freud contributed his part, Klein another part, Lacan another part, although in a different way, of course. And what I risk as a hypothesis is that it contributed *discourse*. Psychoanalysis contributed discourse to heterosexuality.

This in the same sense in which Lacan says that Marx gave discourse to capitalism:

> Lacan says that it was Marx who gave discourse to capitalism, by doing something different with the *obscure function* of surplus value. In this way, the notion of surplus value and the surplus of play are placed in homology; and it will be Lacan who will give discourse to psychoanalysis.

Lacan will say (1968–1969):

> Labour was not new in the production of the commodity, just as the renunciation of jouissance was not new. . . . This renunciation constitutes the master. . . . The novelty is that there is a discourse that articulates this renunciation and makes appear what I will call the function of the plus de jouir, an operation that he locates as the essence of analytic discourse.

Discourse-giving participates in the ambiguous possibility of making another discourse consist of and produce another discourse, a possible way out of the real effects that each discourse produces-provokes.

I hypothesise that psychoanalysis gave discourse to heterosexuality, along with other "disciplines". Obviously, this location of psychoanalysis in the disciplinary is a provocation, but it is not gratuitous. By other disciplines I mean medicine, of course, and in particular psychiatry, in the joint enterprise of biopower and the psi function made visible by Foucault.

There would be a truth of the subject in sex – always said in the masculine. Not without reason, the subject is masculine, thus it was produced by and for men – a truth of sex, a true sex, a truth subject to sex . . . subjection of sex. One could write something called *On Voluntary Sexual Subjection*, paraphrasing La Boétie in *On Voluntary Servitude*, although one would have to problematise the "voluntary" part.

iv.

Very recently, someone in my family who is expecting a child told me that they still don't know the sex and that they can't stand the anxiety any longer, that they might ask to bring the ultrasound scan forward. In the face of which, not without astonishment, I realise how unbearable it is that the sex-generic non-location of that being that arrives in the desire of the parents is. The princeps moment of a binarism that admits no representational ambiguities, a moment in which sexual difference, the religion of the West, the political-visual system, biologic . . . will be summoned and invoked as magic and incantation.

Then a story comes to mind that my mother, a literature teacher and feminist of difference, wrote many years ago, in which she recounted the effects of the disillusionment of a father who, expecting a son, had to register a daughter in the civil registry. He is so disappointed that he forgets the name: Amelia. He disdainfully registers her as Sandalia. To understand the punch line, it is perhaps necessary to say that in the old days, in some places, girls were contemptuously called *chancletas*, a depreciated synonym for sandals.

Even further back in my memories, my first encounter with a trans woman comes to mind. When I was four years old, I went to see Carnival in the city, on the banks of a black river, where I lived. While I was there, I had a revelation: on one of the carriages I saw a woman who appeared imposing to me, like a beautiful and disturbing monster. When I asked my father for her identity, all I got was a reply: "I'll explain later".

I had been baptised in the waters of transgender eros, and my head would never be in its place again. And again my mother, the great fabulator and her tales of small-town characters who defy all normality, all inclusion that is not monstrous:

> At first glance he is a man. His suit is masculine, he wears a tie and buckled shoes, men's socks. And even a hat on her head with a garçon haircut. Despite all this, they call her La cotita, a nickname that is as uncomfortable for her as a dress. . . . She frequented the political clubs of one of the traditional partisan parties when few women dared to mingle with the men. We don't know what life's vagaries led her to bury her feminine condition. I heard that she worked as a labourer on the estancias. On more than one ranch.

She writes *this* and I seem to see it happen and I get that mix of emotions between admiration and embarrassment again.

v.

I was born in 1968, which will certainly not be without consequences. My parents, close to the Tupamaros National Liberation Movement (MNL) since their participation in the March 26th Movement, celebrants of the sexual revolution and David Cooper's *The Death of the Family*, made us all bathe together – children, fathers, mothers, brothers, and sisters – in order to lose our shame in a sort of naïve attempt to naturalise sexual difference and avoid the repression, or at least give it a detour. I, mainly out of shame in front of my sister, who was a year older than me, hid my penis between my legs in a kind of camouflage or concealment – I learned this much later – similar to trans, transvestite, or *drag queen* trickery.

At the age of 16, at the behest of a very close friend, I began an analysis that was to last seven years and which began – at least that is how I remember it, although nothing assures the historical truth of this or any other memory – with a question from the analyst about my relationship with my father. "Well", I said, which made it obvious to that analyst that there was a lot of material to be cut. But, beyond the anecdote that could be analysed, problematised in many ways, what I find interesting today is that it refers to the father. And I don't say *my* father, because I understand that it was something else that would mark me more strongly. What would my relationship to my father be? My pére-version, my father version, my version of the father. (I must say that I began to study French at the age of four at the Alliance Française in my city, which was, moreover, during the Uruguayan dictatorship, a space of freedom and resistance, or at least a refuge for people on the left, so the French signifier game is not alien to me.)

Then came interpretive phenomenological analysis (IPA), which I saw as the only alternative if I wanted to become a psychoanalyst. "The IPA is Freud's institution", it was said . . . His house, his family, one could say, his heirs lived there.

I did my analysis, for fourteen years, two or even three times a week – that was the style – with an IPA analyst. I did supervisions for the time stipulated to apply for admission, I participated in the required study groups, I attended congresses and conferences, etc. I applied for admission and was not admitted. I was not told much about the reasons for non-admission, except something very vague about the aggressiveness, which I still don't know if it was too much or too little, or insufficiently processed, who knows. I was to return to analysis and eventually reapply to be part of Freud's institution, which fortunately I didn't do . . .

At that time, I wrote a humorous and hurt text called: "La ipa no me hizo upa", a text that, once again, I lost, I hid from me, and that today I would like to read. All this not to talk *about* me, but *from* me. Especially today, when it is said that *queer* is theory or activism and that it is necessary to contrast it with psychoanalysis, which is clinical, and that queer theorists don't read, don't know psychoanalysis, and that's why they criticise it.

I'm probably also speaking *from myself*, to make myself one of the recipients of Paul B. Preciado's warm greeting to an improbable mutant in psychoanalysis, on the occasion of his intervention at the 49th Conference of the École de la Cause Freudienne: *Women in psychoanalysis*, on 17 November 2019:

> Good morning, dear ladies, dear gentlemen, of the French School of Psychoanalysts, ladies and gentlemen of the School of the Freudian Cause, and I don't know if it is worth my saying good morning to all those who are neither ladies nor gentlemen, because I don't think there is among you anyone who has legally and publicly renounced sexual difference and who has been accepted as a psychoanalyst . . ., after having successfully passed. I am talking here about a *trans*

> or non-binary psychoanalyst who has been admitted among you. If he exists, let me send that mutant, immediately, the warmest greetings.

May Paul be wrong and may there be, in psychoanalysis, more and more mutants who dare to speak his degenerate name.

vi.

Then came the École Lacanienne de Psychanalyse and its acceptance of *gay and lesbian studies*, a movement, a political gesture that renewed my desire to be part of a school of psychoanalysis. A gesture of welcome that I did not think I would see, having resigned myself to living dissociated in two fields of experience: that of erotics and that of psychoanalysis, irretrievably separated.

As I have already pointed out in *Of a power that is not exercised*, I saluted and still salute today the echo of Jean Allouch (2005), when, as he recounts in his text *Avergonzados*, he experiences a shame that is Jacques Lacan's, his own, and everyone's: and wonders whether he will be authorised to preside over a meeting with trans people and the École Lacanienne de Psychanalyse.

vii.

To conclude, I will say something about how, for me at least, this reception of the degenerate in and by psychoanalysis continues: by importuning it. In a text called *Psychoanalysis as importuned or as a result of disillusionment*, I said:

> In the first session of the seminar *From an Other to the Other*, Lacan declares himself to be importuned by Marx. He does not say concerned, implicated, touched . . . he says importuned, that is to say annoyed, solicited, intervened by, we would say today.

Lacan will allow himself to be intervened, pestered, without this resulting in some kind of ideological subjugation, with consequences for him and his field of practice: psychoanalysis. The result of a traffic between dissimilar fields of knowledge, using homology as an operation and complex language passages, the plus valence will give way to the *plus de jouir*. From this will derive effects for analytical practice: "I will turn to Marx, whose words I have long been bothered by, I regret not having introduced earlier in a field where he is nevertheless perfectly in place" (Lacan, 2008b).

It is not at all obvious that we analysts can do so with what feminisms, queer theory, and decolonialism are importing on psychoanalysis today. What is certain is that we cannot ignore it or deny it by saying "that is not psychoanalysis" anymore. And if we say anymore, it is because we did that for a long time. We did more, I think, we played – without knowing it, knowing that we were doing it – a card of validation of heteronormativity. And I add: "But what are the things psychoanalysis is bothered about?" The answer is so simple as to be absurd: in everything. Surely some Lacanian will remind me of Lacan's not-everything, *pas tout*. So I will sharpen my aim: psychoanalysis is importuned in its non-all. Not because it is necessary to take up some kind of totality – quite the contrary – but because perhaps it is time to review how not-all this not-all is, if it excludes exclusions that constitute and institute it.

I pass review: psychoanalysis has been disturbed[14] by the notions of man, woman, Oedipus, phallus, castration, sexual difference, active-passive, love . . . Is it necessary to continue? And if we were to add the questions posed by decolonial theories or intersectionality: is psychoanalysis a Eurocentric invention from a colonial logos, is there room for something else, what can psychoanalysis say about the racialisation of bodies or poverty and class, what happens not only with its subjective effects but with the very production of the subjective there?

Today I would say, almost without fear of being wrong, for it jumps out at anyone who wants to see, a kind of hard core that resists the degeneration of psychoanalysis and constitutes one of its foundations: sexual difference.

"The rock of castration" is nothing but an effect of this supposal, the basis of all binarism, of all sexuality, of all endosheteronormativity. Preciado (2019b) alludes to this: "the regime of sexual difference, with which psychoanalysis works, is neither a nature nor a symbolic order, but rather a political epistemology of the body, and, as such, is historical and changing". And he adds:

> the regime of sexual difference that you know and consider as universal and quasi-metaphysical, on which all psychoanalytic theories are based and articulated, is neither an empirical reality nor a symbolic order, founder of the unconscious. It is nothing more than *an* epistemology of the living, an anatomical cartography, a political economy of the body and a collective management of this reproductive energy.
>
> It is a historical epistemology that is constructed in relation to a racial taxonomy, as much as to European mercantile and colonial development, and which crystallises in the second half of the nineteenth century.
>
> This epistemology, far from being the representation of a reality, is a performative machine that produces and legitimises a specific political and economic order: hetero-colonial patriarchy.

Already in *An Apartment on Uranus. Crónicas del cruce*, he had written: "If the heteropatriarchal regime of sexual difference is the scientific religion of the West, then changing sex cannot be anything but a heretical act" (Preciado, 2019b). Sexual difference is the scientific religion of the West. Visual-political regime. Something similar, though put differently, Oyeronké Oyewumi (2017) will point out in *The Invention of Women*. Bio-logic, she will call it.

I salute the wisdom of Leo Bersani (2011) when in *The Freudian Body. Psychoanalysis and art* he points out that "we address theoretical texts insofar as *their theoretical position fails in the formulation*" making truth and failure, truth and "theoretical lapse" in Freud absolutely supportive.

It is enough to reread *Some Psychical Consequences of the Anatomical Difference of the Sexes* (Freud, 1986b) to see the *epistemology* referred to by Preciado and others. However, there is an inconsistent coexistence between a naturalisation of sexual difference as an extra-linguistic a priori in tension with the impossibility of making it a scientific fact:

> [T]he little girl. She notices the penis of a brother or a little playmate, a penis that is clearly visible and of non-table size, and at once discerns it as the corresponding, superior, of her own small, hidden organ; thereupon she falls victim to penis envy. . . . In the analogous case, when the little boy sees the genital region of the girl for the first time, he is irresolute, uninterested at first; he sees nothing, or denies his perception, he deludes it, he seeks subterfuges to make it conform to his expectation. Only later, after a threat of castration has gained influence over him, will that observation become significant for him; its recollection or renewal stirs in him a fearful affective storm, and subjects him to the belief in the effectiveness of the threat which he had hitherto laughed at.
>
> (Freud, 1986b)

Or further on: "The difference between male and female in this part of sexual development is an understandable consequence of the anatomical diversity of the genitalia and of the psychical situation connected with it (Freud, 1986b). And a little more:

> We will not allow ourselves to be misled by the objections of the faith-minists who want to impose on us a complete equalisation and identical appreciation of the two sexes; but we will willingly conceive that the majority of men also lag far behind the male ideal, and that all human individuals, as a result of their bisexual (constitutional) disposition and cross-inheritance, combine male and female characters, so that pure masculinity and femininity remain theoretical constructions of uncertain content.

Already at that time, feminists were making this political reification of difference an obstacle, to which we pay tribute. Bersani calls this always unsuccessful attempt to theoretically stabilise psychoanalytical findings "domesticating clarities of narrative orders".

In *Psychoanalysis an erotology of passage*, Jean Allouch (1998) says, again, something that seems to me fundamental: psychoanalysis will be an erotology of passage if it succeeds in abandoning "the man-woman partition". If and only if . . . I say. In this sense, something seems to be opening up since the emphasis that Allouch (2017) has been placing for some time now on Lacan's "there is no sexual relation". Something that, to my way of thinking, would make it possible to leave behind the notion of castration and, probably, of lack. The non-existence of sexual relation, in the mathematical sense of writing, radicalises the logical impossibility of heterosexuality hitherto seen as obligatory or destiny.

However, it is not evident to me that it means dropping sexual difference, resulting from the sex-gender binarism as a system (Rubin, 1975), unless we conclude that there is no sexual relation because *there is no sexual*. Unless we stop regulating ourselves by difference and do so by the diverse and multiple. Non-existence of the sexual relation that is also in the same act *non-existence of the sexual*, not to be *conquered* (I don't like any conquest). I am more seduced by saying: non-existence to be *realised* (playing with the real and the realisation).

Let's leave it here, at least for now . . .

On androgenesis in a case of female homosexuality or heterosexuality as destiny

i. By way of excuse

Some time ago, in *Zona clínica degenerada, a* collective of cross-readings in feminisms, queer theory, and psychoanalysis, we set out to reread cases of psychoanalysis from the perspective of contemporary feminist warnings.

On the occasion of revisiting the so-called Dora case (Freud, 1905), together with the collective *Zona clínica degenerada*, we noted once again the permanent oscillations in Freudian discourse between what Leo Bersani (2011) points out as the highly speculative and novelty of Freudian discovery-invention and the "normalising orders" of his discourse.

This meant that psychoanalysis missed its historical opportunity not to contribute to the *dispositif of sexuality*, the *sex-gender system*, and *heterosexuality as a political regime*.

Gayle Rubin (1975) will also say this in her own way:

> Psychoanalysis offers a description of the mechanisms by which the sexes are divided and deformed, and how androgynous and bisexual children are transformed into boys and girls. Psychoanalysis is a frustrated feminist theory.

After revisiting Dora, we continued with *On the Psychogenesis of a Case of Female Homosexuality*, from 1920 (Freud, 1905). The bet was to reread it with what Lacan had commented on and reformulated in his seminars, with the book by Inés Rieder and Diana Voigt (2004), *Sidonie Csilag. Freud's Young Homosexual Girl*, and with Jean Allouch's *The Shadow of Your Dog* (2004) and his proposal of an erotic doggerie, an erotics of dog-love at play there. However, the impact of Freud's rereading on his invention of the case was enough to precipitate what I will try to argue as follows.

Judith Butler (2007) says in *Gender in Dispute* that Oedipus in its two versions – positive and negative – enables nothing but heterosexuality. One desires the mother as a male and one desires the father as a woman, independently of gender assignment. These are positions that in Freud appear to be linked to the anatomical difference of the sexes, from which only one destiny, the heterosexual, seems possible.

> The notion of bisexuality as *dispositions* – female and male – that have heterosexual goals as intentional correlates makes it clear that for Freud *bisexuality is the coincidence of two heterosexual desires within a single psyche*. In reality, the male disposition is never oriented towards the father as the object of sexual love, nor is the female disposition oriented towards the mother (the girl may have such a disposition, but this occurs before she has renounced that "masculine" side of her natural disposition). By rejecting the mother as the object of sexual love, the girl necessarily rejects her masculinity and paradoxically "establishes" her femininity as a consequence. Thus, in Freud's thesis of primary bisexuality there is no homosexuality and only opposites attract.

Heterosexuality is destiny.

Right from the start, Freud – not without half warning – shows the threads of his invention and its political consequences. Politics that will not be reduced to a politics of psychoanalysis but to psychoanalysis as a politics of the sexual.

James Strachey says, on the subject of "On the psychogenesis of a case of female homosexuality":

> If in the "Dora" case (1905e) [1901]), and in his contributions to *Studies on Hysteria* (1895d), he had dealt almost exclusively with hysteria, he now began to consider in greater depth the whole question of sexuality in women. His research in this area would later lead him to write his works on the anatomical difference between the sexes (1925j) and on female sexuality (1931b), as well as his *New Introductory Lectures on Psychoanalysis* (1933a). The present article also contains an account of some of Freud's later conceptions of homosexuality in general.
>
> (Freud, 1989a)

In this framework, the case of the so-called homosexual girl seeks to confirm her previous speculations from the clinic. Just as one seeks to locate a truth of the subject in sex, the clinic would be the place of a truth of theory, and this would then be an unnoticed epistemic-political option.

Freud (1989c) says:

> Female homosexuality, indeed as frequent as male homosexuality, if much less strident, has not only escaped criminal law; it has also been neglected by psychoanalytic research. For this reason, it is perhaps worth considering the communication of a single, and not too flagrant, case in which the history of its psychic genesis could be recorded almost without gaps and with complete certainty.

Putting criminal investigation and psychoanalysis in the same sentence cannot fail to trigger in me somewhat persecutory concerns, but I will allow them to be foisted on me on account of my paranoia.

Secondly, lesbian invisibility is taken as a given, unproblematised, and even used as a justification for resorting to the single case as evidence. The same will happen with "women" and so-called "female sexuality" or the Oedipus in women, in the absence of greater knowledge – or on account of a lack of knowledge of what is (in)made visible as a *dark continent* – I think it is not necessary to underline the racist implications of this mode of enunciation – the "feminine" will again come out of the rib of the masculine.

ii. The sayings made

The case is presented to us:

> An eighteen-year-old girl, beautiful and intelligent, from a family of high social standing, provokes the displeasure and care of her parents by the tenderness with which she pursues a "society" lady, ten years older than herself. The parents claim that this lady, despite her aristocratic surname, is nothing more than a *cocotte*. They say they know that she lives in the house of a close friend with whom she has intimate relations, while at the same time indulging in dissolute love affairs with a number of men. The girl does not question this bad reputation, but this does not deter her from her adoration for the lady, even though she has no lack of sense of propriety and propriety. She is not deterred by any prohibition or vigilance from taking advantage of the rare occasions to be in the company of her beloved, to spy on all her habits of life, to wait for her for hours and hours at the door of her house or at the tram stop, to send her flowers, and so on.

The case is presented to us not without considerations:

> It is evident that this one interest has devoured all others in the girl. She does not care to continue her education, she attaches no value to social intercourse or to the entertainments proper to young girls, and only keeps in touch with a few friends who may serve as confidants or helpers. The parents do not know how far things have gone between their daughter and this dubious lady, and whether they have gone beyond the limits of tender enthusiasm. They have never noticed that the girl was interested in young men and was pleased by their compliments; on the other hand, they are well aware that she has been in love with a young man.
>
> It is clear that this present inclination towards a woman only continues to an extreme extent what in recent years had been insinuated towards persons of the female sex and had aroused the father's anger and rigour.

If *Hitting a child* could be the phrase of a ghost, *Makes the father angry* or even, as I will show later: *Cheats the father*, *Takes revenge on the father*, could be the phrases of this Freudian ghost. Something has gone beyond a certain family limit, it has reached an extreme, it has become intolerable. The family is political. And the intolerable that goes beyond the familiar appeals to psychoanalysis, which, although Freud says "discredited', seems to offer a certain expectation of normalisation, of a return to the mainstream.

It is here that Freud seems to oscillate, once again, between a lucid acceptance of the political demand for psychoanalysis and its inappropriateness, and an assent for the sake of the disciplinary construction of a knowledge that seeks the signifiers of its recognition:

> I was not faced with the situation which analysis demands, and the only one in which it can demonstrate its efficacy. This situation, as is well known, in the fullness of its ideal notes, presents the following aspect: someone, in the most self-possessed state, suffers from an inner conflict which he cannot put an end to on his own; he then goes to the analyst, formulates his complaint and asks for his help. The doctor then works side by side with a part of the personality split in two by the illness, and against the other party to the conflict. Situations that deviate from these are more or less unfavourable for the analysis, and add new difficulties to those intrinsic to the case. Situations such as those of the building contractor who commissions the architect to build a house according to his taste and needs, or the pious donor who has a sacred image painted by the artist, in a corner of which his own portrait in the form of an adorer then finds its place, are fundamentally not compatible with the conditions of psychoanalysis. . . . In short, it makes no difference whether an individual comes to analysis out of his own desire or because others have brought him to it; whether he himself wishes to change or only his friends want this change; whether he wants to change or not; whether he wants to change himself or only his friends want to change. The people close to him, the people who love him or from whom this love should be expected.

He even states:

> The girl was not a sick person – she was not suffering from internal razones or complaining about her condition, and the task at hand was not to solve a neurotic conflict, but to transfer one variant of the sexual genital organisation to another.

The question seems unavoidable: why initiate an analysis at all, and who benefits from this attempt? And no less important, who is/were harmed by it?

Jean Allouch (2005) says in "Ashamed": "We have Freud's soul and our theory confirmed. It is easily overlooked, that, elsewhere, without our even knowing it, thank God, the broken dishes will be paid for, the price will be paid".

Freud seems to justify himself:

> For these reasons, I avoided altogether painting to the parents the prospect of their wish being fulfilled. I merely declared myself ready to study the girl carefully for a few weeks or months, in order to be able to pronounce afterwards on the chances of obtaining any effect by further analysis.

iii. Of adoptions, delegations, and abandonments

The delegation to other fields of the political decisions of psychoanalysis produces nothing but political effects. Let us look at some of this with regard to the status of the masculine and the feminine:

> Psychoanalysis stands on common ground with biology insofar as it adopts as its premise an originary bisexuality of the human individual (so as of the animal). But he cannot elucidate the essence of that which in the conventional or biological sense is called "masculine" and "feminine"; he *adopts both concepts and bases his work on them.*
>
> (Freud, 1986b) (Italics are mine)

What is the cost of this adoption? Or on homosexuality:

> It is not the mission of psychoanalysis to solve the problem of homosexuality. It has to be content with revealing the psychic mechanisms that have led to the choice of object, and from there to trace the paths that lead to the drive dispositions. At that point he ceases his task and abandons the rest to biological research.
>
> (Freud, 1986b)

Adoptions, delegations, abandonments that not only affect analytic theory and practice but also produce it. Freud does not rule out a *therapy of inversion* either – he only considers that it is still too hasty to think about it, except in cases of marked symatic hermaphroditism: "Nevertheless, it would be haste or harmful exaggeration to cherish the hope of a 'therapy' of inversion that would be universally applicable" (Freud, 1986b).

But let us return to the so-called homosexual girl, from whom Freud seeks to obtain "an overview of the forces that transported the girl's libido from the normal Oedipal attitude to that of homosexuality, as well as the psychic paths that were transferred for this", i.e., the psychogenesis of the case.

As in Dora, despite positing constitutional or original bisexuality as an innate and universal human disposition, Freud does not cease to posit the existence of a normal Oedipus:

> "The girl had gone through her infantile years, in an unremarkable way, with the normal attitude of the female Oedipus complex".

The analysis then gives rise to a hermeneutic of whose textual basis we know nothing – we do not have the young woman's sayings – only supposed facts and their interpretation or *inference*:

> Between the ages of thirteen and fourteen he showed a tender and, in everyone's opinion, exaggerated predilection for a little boy who had not yet reached the

> age of three and whom he could see regularly in a playground. So much did he take the child to heart that a long-standing friendly relationship with the child's parents was born out of it. From this *it can be inferred* that at that time she was dominated by a strong desire to become a mother herself and have a child. But soon afterwards the child began to be indifferent to her, and she began to show an interest in older, though still young, women, an interest whose exteriorisations soon brought her a heartfelt reprimand from the father.
>
> (Freud, 1986) (Italics are mine)

And he adds: "Before, her libido had been directed towards her mother; afterwards she was a homosexual in love with more mature women, as she continued to be thereafter". Then came an event that Freud describes as an event: "a new pregnancy of the mother and the birth of a third brother when she was sixteen years old".

Without interruption, Freud goes on to unveil the synthesis of his analysis, with a single caveat that seeks to allay suspicions about the implementation of what he calls "his combinatorial gifts":

> The plot that I am about to reveal in what follows is not the product of some combinatorial gifts that I would have; it was suggested to me by analytic material so trustworthy that I can claim for it an objective certainty.

Don't clarify that obscures, we would say today. And a list of "revelations" goes on and on:

> The beloved lady was a substitute for . . . the mother/ "The slim silhouette, the dour beauty and the rough character of the lady reminded him of her.

Therefore, the object ultimately chosen corresponded not only to her ideal of a woman, but also to her ideal of a man; it brought together the satisfaction of the two orientations of desire, the homosexual and the heterosexual

> /the mother relegates her behind the brothers and seeks to distance her from the father/disappointed by the mother she will seek a child from the father, a child which she not only does not obtain but which is given to her competitor, the mother/she will then turn her back on the father and on men in general and turn to women, thus leaving the way open to the mother/ "she disregarded her femininity and sought another placement for her libido", "she has rejected her femininity and sought another placement for her libido".
>
> (Freud, 1989c)

Here begins what I will call *Freud's androgenic operation*, resulting from the application of male "libidinal development" to this "inverted" woman. It thus produces an equivalence: a homosexual woman is the same as a heterosexual man, only in a female body.

The woman does not exist.

Let us look at some indications of what I am saying. Regarding the disillusionment with the father, who gives a child to the mother and not to her, he will say:

> Thus he behaved in all things like many men, who, after a first painful experience, make a lasting break with the feminised sex of women and become misogynists.

The "new occupation of her libido" will correspond with the assumption of a masculine type of object choice and even with a masculine model of love for women, courtly love, the young heterosexual girl will become *a gentleman*: "she changed into a man and took the mother in the place of the father as an object of love".

The explanation is given:

> I have said that the girl adopted in relation to the revered lady the *masculine type of love*. Her humiliation. *His* happiness when he was allowed to accompany the lady a little longer and to kiss her hand at parting; his delight when her beauty was praised, while he was not a whit ashamed that third parties should recognise his own beauty; his pilgrimage to places where the beloved had once resided; the silencing of the most daring sensual desires: these are so many other *small traits which perhaps contribute to the first passionate enthusiasm of a young man for a famous artist* whom he believes to be far above him and to whom, self-conscious, he hardly dares to raise his gaze. The coincidence with a "masculine type of object choice", described by me and whose peculiarities I had traced back to the link with the mother, went right down to the details.
>
> (Freud, 1986) (Italics are mine)

And how could one explain the attraction for a lady of such a bad reputation as the one who gave rise to this outburst? *If your only tool is a hammer, you will only see a nail in every problem*, as the saying goes: "the whole enigma of this behaviour is dispelled if we remember that also for that masculine type of object choice, derived from the mother, there is the condition that the beloved has in some way a 'bad sexual reputation'".

In *On a particular type of object choice in man (Contributions to the psychology of love)* of 1910, he had said that there were two conditions for this love. The first, which he will call: the condition of the "injured third party".

> . . . its content is that the person in question never chooses as an object of love a woman who remains free, that is, a lady or a lady who is alone, but always one over whom another man can claim property rights.
>
> (Freud, 1989a)

And the second condition:

> that the chaste and unsuspicious woman never exercises the attraction that can elevate her to an object of love, but only one whose sexual conduct in any way deserves a bad reputation, and whose fidelity and character are of the highest quality. and whose fidelity and blameless character may be doubted.
>
> (Freud, 1989a)

Derived from doubts about the virginal character of the mother, this virgin/whore division: "The enquiry then takes us back to the time of life when the little boy first had more complete knowledge of the sexual relations between his parents".

And what in this earlier paper was part of the male master's life is now, ten years later, transposed to the young homosexual girl, who has become a "little man". This is confirmed by Strachey's footnote: "In a paper written several years later, 'On the psychogenesis of a case of female homosexuality', Freud proved the existence of the same type of object choice in a homosexual girl".

Lacan will point out Freud's confusion about the imaginary transference and the symbolic transference, about the passage to the act as the effect of the subject's encounter with the object, in the seminars *The Object Relationship* and *Anguish*. And he will make of the young homosexual girl a *courteous lover*. Jean Allouch (2004), in *The shadow of your dog*, will construct from the case, clarified by the research of Ines Rieder and Diana Voigt (2004), a new erotic figure: the dog-love and a mastery – making the young homosexual girl a Master, which does not cease to pose problems for us.

However, there has not yet been a subjective rectification, which would be at the same time political, of Freud's androgenising operation. Perhaps it is not up to me to do it either – even if I felt qualified to do so – but to the lesbian theorists, while we continue to listen to the words – transcribed by the biographers of the so-called young homosexual – that the no-longer-young analysand dedicated to us:

> On the other side of the street, to the left and right of the Palais Caprara-Geymüller portal, two Atlanteans are struggling to carry the weight of the world on their shoulders, their gaze as stony and desperate as if it were all the evils of the world.
>
> The two Atlanteans are struggling to carry the weight of the world on their shoulders, their gaze as stony and despairing as if they were carrying all the world's ills. Until now he had not noticed these figures, but that is precisely how it feels at Freud's . . . it is unbearable.
>
> (Rieder and Voigt, 2004)

She will then try to "get out of the mess" and, if possible, convince her father to allow her to finish her analysis. She, at least, has already completed it internally and dreams of the south (Rieder and Voigt).

Freud interrupted the treatment, suspecting the young woman's deception, by means of dreams in which she longed for: "the cure of the investment by the treatment, expressed her joy at the prospects of life now open to her, confessed her longing for the love of a man and for children" (Freud, 1986).

The young woman seeks to deceive him, like her father. He will have to refer her to a female analyst in order to overcome the transferential obstacle.

> I told her one day that I did not believe these dreams, that they were mendacious or hypocritical and that she intended to deceive me as she used to deceive her father. I was not wrong; the dreams of that kind ceased after that hiding. However, I believe that along with the purpose of misleading me there was also a hint of courtship in these dreams; it was also an attempt to win my interest and my good nature, perhaps in order to disappoint me later in greater depth.
>
> (Freud, 1986)

The case closes in a verbal act of Freud's, which sheds even more light, if that is possible, on what was at stake there, in that (mis)encounter:

> When Freud, at the first session after the summer, informs her of his decision, Sidonie is inwardly relieved. She had complied with the forms and had shown her father that she had shown goodwill. But then again, not everything can be changed. If Professor Freud communicates this to her father and adds that Leonie never took her away from her father.
>
> That Leonie never pushed her out of the way by taking her to his bed, he will stay calm and leave her alone. Thus everything has once again taken the best possible course for her. At parting, Professor Freud says to her:
>
> "You have such intelligent eyes. I would not want to meet you as an enemy in my life".
>
> (Rieder and Voigt, 2004)

What about this Freudian witticism, what about the fear and persecution of an intelligent, non-heterosexual woman, what about the paranoid – which Freud had linked to homosexuality in the Schreber case – seems to be reversed in the professor's case?

On the affects as the politics of the subjective

i. Of performance and affects

In *How to be Gay*, David Halperin (2015) made me open my eyes to a fact that – for a change – I always knew without knowing it: there *are* no *affects*. There is a politics of affects, a dramaturgy and hegemonic practices, Eurocentric, heteronormative, class and race, etc., that matrix the ways in which we affect ourselves and that which affects us. It is a matrix that makes affects a place of subjective truth, denying them any performative and political character. For this matrix, there would be only one way of experiencing what we call grief, sadness, joy, pain, etc. The *queer* experience disproves this supposed universality or *affective normativity*. The multiple, parodic, performative ways in which the gay community dealt with the AIDS pandemic are just one demonstration of this.

So there is no longer a single way of dealing with it.

Halperin asks: *What are drag queens laughing about?* As an example, he refers to the so-called Long Island Widows, gay men who lost their partners to AIDS, who perform a mourning act – or should I say, perform their mourning parodically:

> Fire Island widows laugh first and foremost at their own grief. When they laugh at grisly or tragic situations, it is not that they are oblivious to the horror or tragedy involved – quite the contrary. They laugh so as not to cry, so as not to fall into maudlin self-pity. But that is not all, for the grief does not disappear when they laugh at it, if anything it becomes more acute, more concrete. However, it is thus confined to a known area, a specific social and emotional location, which means that it becomes less constricting, less isolating. Consequently, one does not escape from grief, but shares it in a way that allows one to cope with it.
>
> (Halperin, 2015)

He adds:

> To use one's own grief as a tool of humor, to refuse to exempt oneself from the irony with which one regards all other social identities and personifications of accepted social roles, is, in effect to level social differences . . . not to pretend to be taken seriously and to renounce the right to the empathy of others, to sentimentality.

As Laurent Berlant, Nicolás Cuello, Mariela Solana, Ann Cvetkovich, Sara Ahmed, and many others have pointed out – from differential biases in each case – there is a political dimension of affects or, as I prefer to say, a *political economy of affects* made invisible by this heterosexual, bourgeois, white, Eurocentric-colonial matrix.

On the other hand, as Helena López (Ahmed, 2015) points out in the Prologue to Sara Ahmed's *La política cultural de las emociones*, it will be a matter of resisting a certain queer voluntarism, which I will call naïve not to anchor myself in a determinism but to include potency and diminution of potency, possibility and impossibility, in our existences in multiple affectations. We exist in affectation and affecting.

No longer from the affective turn but from a critical queer perspective, Javier Saez (2015) launched his Molotov bomb some time ago: "Love is heterosexual", which earned him enmity and aggression even from friends and fellow activists.

Saez says:

> I wonder if the rhetoric of love is just another discourse and another practice that we have adopted from the heterosexual regime. In any case, it is a totally harmless and domesticated discourse, something that does not bother the patriarchal

> and homophobic system at all. On the contrary, buns, queers and even trans people are much better digested and accepted when they have pareja ("what healthy boys, they are no longer promiscuous") and especially when they proclaim "their love for each other".

Nor did Jean Genet ([1949] 1976) make good press for himself by affirming *betrayal* as the greatest act of love, when he slept with the Nazi "killer" of his beloved, in a kind of radical asceticism of love. Betrayal: this abject act that is removed from any heroic cause. Can we ask ourselves, for example, whether it is still possible today to maintain that "anguish is the only affection that does not deceive"? And if so, should we conclude that the other affections do deceive? Or perhaps it would be better to say that they perform "something", do "something", seek to affect?

Emotions produce bodies: "bodies take just the form of the contact they have with objects and with others", Sara Ahmed (2015) points out. And she goes further: they shape "the surface of individual and collective bodies". It is a matter of de-subalternating the "surface" with respect to some depth, background, or essence. We are bodies of surface, surface of bodies that affect each other.

And of course, it is also a reaction to a certain structuralism, a certain linguistic turn and a certain psychoanalysis of the hegemony of the symbolic (the product of a political reading of a Lacan untied from his RSI records).

George Didi-Huberman (2016) in *What emotion! What emotion?* recovers the astonishment – as a philosophical gesture – in the face of emotion, as a first step towards critically situating oneself in relation to it. It is precisely Huberman who will highlight emotion as *experience and intensity*. And in a rapid genealogical gesture, he places readers before a Charles Darwin who, in *The Expression of the Emotions in Man and Animals*, situates the emotions as something primitive, more characteristic of the human race.

Finally, Huberman calls into crisis the notion of the radically singular or personal nature of emotions and makes them the effect of a relationship to others. The one who is moved by others, exposes himself, "exposes his powerlessness", says the author, his weakness, while repeating old ways of being affected; a *collective dimension* makes it at a certain point "the emotions of all in each other".

Moreover, the philosopher dissociates emotion from pathos as passive *suffering*, making visible the active character that moves and seeks to move. Emotion, then, as a commotion and motion that transforms, makes the one who experiences it come out of himself. For Huberman, it is more a matter of the order of the *event* than of an egoic or even singular event.

ii. Of affects, effects, and signs

In Lacan, affects as the effect of language on the body, anguish as evidence – a sign of a real there, not as a revelation of being or truth – or at any rate as a sign of the truth of the *sujetx*; affect: "unmoored, drifting. One finds it displaced, mad, inverted, metabolised" (Lacan [1962–3] 2006b). Thought will be for Lacan almost an affect: "Thought is not a category. I would almost say that it is an affect. If only to say that it is the most fundamental thing under the angle of affect", he states in *The Reverse of Psychoanalysis* (Lacan [1969–70] 1992). In *Tele-vision*, he will say: "the affect comes to a body whose peculiarity consists in inhabiting language" (Lacan [1972] 2012b).

But is it enough? Lacan undoubtedly produces a de-naturalisation of affect, understood as reaction or response, making it subsidiary to language, the effect of language and, finally, as a sign of the *real unconscious*, a formulation I prefer to the real unconscious.[15]

Shame – not in its sexual dimension but as a sign of the lack in being – will have a special place for Lacan, being even the affect from which an ethics that he will call *vergonzology* could be underpinned.[16]

However, my hypothesis is that something escapes here from the social, collective, ideal and moral, performative-political dimension of affects. Shame will not be the same for those who inhabit hegemonic bodies and erotics, in accordance with a sex-gender system and a dispositif of sexuality, as it will be for those who transit forms of sex-gender dissidence, or inhabit poverty or racialisation. Nor will it be the same for those who have been designated *men* or those who have been designated *women*. It is about power relations that permeate bodies and discourses with the consequent effects.

Injury constitutes, produces the *sujetx minoritarix*, the *subalternx*, says Didier Eribon (2017), and Édouard Louis (2019) shows it in *Para acabar con Eddy Bellegueulle*.

Eribon says that his sentence "In the beginning was injustice", with which he opens *Identities. Reflections on the gay question* (2001), derives from what he learned with Jean Genet: "someone says to Genet: You are a thief, and Genet makes this name his own, which is thrown over him like a net: I will be the thief". 'The insults followed the blows, and my silence always', says Édouard Louis.

Perhaps a chapter should be written on *loneliness*, as an affect-effect of the discourses of hate, rejection, and exclusion. Tolerable, even enjoyable, solitude is a luxury that not everyone can afford. It will not be the same solitude, even if the signifier belies the difference, that of those on whom it was imposed as a punishment for their abnormality or deviance.

iii. Of happy fragilities

But it is not only about sad affections.

Sara Ahmed (2019) posits happiness as "the unofficial religion of contemporary capitalist society that makes us believe that the possibility of being whatever we want is in the power of each individual"; happiness that in neoliberalism is only in relation to the economic, also denying differences and equalising very unequal lives.

Economic happiness, happiness of the economy? . . . Economics of happiness.

Already in *Queer Fragility*, Ahmed (2018) stated:

> In older uses of queer in the English language – that is, queer to describe that which is striking because it is strange – the concepts queer and fragility were often companions. A companion is a fellow traveller. In one of George Eliot's essays, "Three Months in Weimar", the narrating instance describes the sound of an old piano in this way: "its sounds are now as queer and faint as those of an old invalid woman whose voice might once have made a heart beat with impetuous passion". So: queer and weak. Weak, delicate, invalidx, incapacitate, flinch, faint-hearted, weepy, raídx; desagarrarx; deteriorate; *queer* too, the queer resonates in these words as well. These proximities in meaning tell us a story. We can come into contact with things at the very moment when they are, or we are, worn out or worn down; those moments when we are broken or sinking, when we are shattered under the weight of history.

The author recalls that: "For Eve Kosofsky Sedgwick, what makes *queer a 'term with political potential'* is the way it clings to and refers back to 'scenes of shame from childhood". Already in Willful Subjects (2014), whose translation could be *Willful Subjects*, Ahmed described *awkwardness* as:

> a *queer* ethics. Awkwardness is both a crip ethic and a queer ethic; we have to create spaces for bodies that do not obey orders; that do not move in *straight lines*, that lose their balance. A body that is less stable is less supported by a ground that will, in turn, be less stable for the body. If a world is organised in straight lines, if we have only narrow spaces to move in (e.g., along a corridor or between that table and that window), if tools are made only for hands that can grasp things tightly, consequently activities will be harder to complete for some than for others. Certain activities can make you learn by putting you up against a wall. A wiggling body (wiggles): that deviates from the socially accepted path. Awkwardness: when a world is what you stumble against.

In *Queer Phenomenology* (2006), I had characterised *queer* from the notion of *disorientation*, resulting from: "an oblique or oblique relationship with a straight/heteronormative world" (Ahmed, 2018). The author speaks of *defence* against the heteronormative; I prefer to speak of *subaltern strategies:*

> Building from ruin; our building may appear to be in ruins, when we build, we ruin. How easy, however, without foundations, without a stable floor, for the walls to fall down. We support them; we support each other. So we might think of fragility not so much as the potential to lose something, fragility as loss, but as a quality of relations we acquire or a quality of the building we construct . . . fragility not so much as the potential to lose something, fragility as loss, but as a quality of relations we acquire or a quality of the building we construct.
>
> Queer fragility: a quality of what is built. A fragile shelter has looser walls, made of lighter materials; look how they move; it's a movement.

In *Reflexiones sobre el giro afectivo en historia queer*, Mariela Solana (2016) draws on Elizabeth Freeman, Carolyn Dinshaw, and Heather Love, historians, pioneers of the affective turn in the queer field, who take a very particular slant on the subject: "the way in which the affects of the present can motivate and enrich the study of the past", that is, that they assign epistemic value to affects in the knowledge of history.

Elizabeth Freeman goes so far as to coin the term *erotohistoriography*:

> to foreground the pleasures that can emerge from the encounter with the past (. . .) the emotive, felt and even erotic dimension of the relationship between past and present appears as an unavoidable element in the development of alternative historical narratives about dissident sexuality.

Carolyn Dinshaw rereads Michel Foucault, who,

> . . . despite being considered the great exponent of historical alterism,[17] he admits to being "touched" by the infamous men he finds in his archive. In *The Lives of Infamous Men (*1996), Foucault speaks of a "vibration" he felt when studying these singular and abject lives of the past and how the fragments he found gave him a physical impression and an intensity that is difficult to reconstruct by means of historical writing. Thus, despite maintaining that there is a radical alterity with the past, Foucault re-knows how to feel a connection, a way of vibrating with those men, however impossible this might seem.

The effects of the injury that constitutes the dissident *sujetx*, that subjectively produces it, is only found again in resonance with those who come into contact with that story, with those who read that life. However, this will not be enough to create a community in identification. With regard to Dinshaw, Solana states that:

> echoes Halperin's definition of queer as an identity that does not have a positive essence but is a position in relation to norms. This allows the author to compose "a queer history without the mechanisms of identification, similarity or filiation. This connection is made possible not by a shared identity but by a shared solitude. This is an oxymoron, as is the queer community".

For a long time, we subaltern subjects have been talked about, theorised, objectified, and subjectivised by others who, from positions of privilege, thought it necessary to highlight the deviation from the normal in order to make exceptions the justification for the rule.

Today we are spoken by others, often with a paternalistic understanding. However, for some time now, we monsters have been speaking out, and I don't believe that they will silence us, or that we will be silenced.

Return of the oppressed.

Deleuze-Guattari, a queer-degenerate *machine*

Although Michel Foucault's influence on the propitiation of the conditions of discursive possibility of the queer field is more widely recognised than that of Deleuze-Guattari, this fact does not seem to me to be entirely fair.

It is undeniable that the Foucauldian discourse of non-discourse as a device of sexuality and its problematisation of the relation of the subject to the apparatuses of veridiction, as well as the historical construction of abnormality, madness, homosexuality, etc., constitutes one of the foundations on which the queer-dissident wager is based.

In the Deleuze-Guattari machine, it is a machinic agency that produces effects through its composition. I will maintain this way of naming this scriptural and discursive agency, making my own Leonor Silvestri's (2020) apt description of what constitutes today a queer-degenerate discursivity. It will not only be a matter of contents, notions, or concepts – in the sense that Deleuze gives to this term – the concept is not without the creation-invention of conceptual characters, intrinsic presences, the condition of positivity of thought itself. Even if it were only a matter of notions: becomings, deterritorialisation, body without organs, machinic agency, and so many others, they would be enough to recognise this opening up of other ways of rethinking the subjective. And if it is a question of anti-recognitions, let us at least mention Spinoza. Anti-recognition is an ironic formulation that questions the notion of recognition. Spinoza is the one who enables agency as much as the capacity to "compose" with everything that increases our powers, which enables multiple agency, monsters, etc., as the great proto-queer in this improbable genealogy.

Very recently, and in the wake of the so-called affective turn, Wen Liu (2020), of the University of Albany (New York), attempted a promising articulation in "Feeling dejected, regressive and machinic: queer theory and the affective turn". Articulation, crossing of notions that I will not analyse here but that I am interested in mentioning as a sign of the validity of reconsidering the contributions of this writing machine that came to be called Deleuze-Guattari.

By way of illustration, Wen Liu there sets out what he calls "three distinct but related *strains* of works of affect: queer negativity, queer temporality and the queer as machinic body" (a disturbing term in this pandemic context). The machinic will then open up as one of the ways of understanding modes of affect, as well as a platform for enabling notions such as prosthetic body, techno-body, and so on.

Guy Hocquenghem, in *Homosexual Desire* ([1972] 2009), was one of the first to see this deviant potential of the *Anti-Oedipus*. Thus, for example, with regard to anal eroticism, he will say:

> Only the spirit is capable of shitting. Deleuze and Guattari's phrase is understood in the sense that only the spirit is capable of fabricating the excremental, only sublimations are capable of situating the anal. Between the summits where

> the spirit blows and the underworld of the anus, between the sublime and the excremental, our anal sexuality is enclosed.

Many years later, Nestor Perlongher (1991), from another geopolitical context and other theoretical-activist directions, would also draw on the Deleuzo-Guattarian discourse.

> Becoming is molecular, it mobilises particles in turbulence by extracting them from the great molar oppositions. Where there were only two great molar sexes (you will be A or B, you will be a man or a woman), a thousand small molecular sexes, in the empire of sensation, in the intensive. From the woman as a molar identity captured in the binary opposition of the "total" sexes, a kind of "micro-femineity" emerges: it is a question of "producing in ourselves the molecular woman, creating the molecular woman".

In 1981, moreover, Perlongher introduced Guattari during his stay in Brazil. Something similar, though different, happened in 1982 with Pedro Lemebel during Guattari's stay in Chile.

Perlongher's *neobarroso* and Lemebel's *neobarrocho* find appropriable echoes in this baroque machine, if we agree with José Javier Maristany's proposal (2008): "It would not be risky to think of his *Mil mesetas* as a finished exponent of the neo-baroque, both in its conception as a book and in its writing, and thus turn the sense of flows and appropriations upside down".

Let us listen to some of what Lemebel (2000) says in *Loco afán, Crónicas de sidario:*

> From a ligoso imaginary I expel these excedent materials to disguise political desire in oppression. I become a beetle that weaves its black honey, I become a woman like any other minority. I indulge in its matrix of outrage, I make alliances with the indolatine mother, and I learn the patriarchal language to curse her.

With regard to the neo-baroque (neo-baroque soiled by the river Mapocho), let me recommend Soledad Bianchi's article (2015): *Del neobarroco o la inestabilidad del taco alto.*

So, let's make a second anti-recognition here, just by naming two major queers of this improbable genealogy: Severo Sarduy and Lezama Lima.

Perhaps my queer nomination for this discursive machine derives from how I understand queer along the lines of David Halperin (2015) in *How to be Gay:* a deviant vocation, a desire to twist everything, to invert everything, everything that is claimed to be straight, including the straight, which is no tomb but for compulsory heterosexuality.

Halperin describes this appropriating and deviant wager in different ways:

> Gay culture[18] generates and elaborates a specific sensibility and a singular way of relating to the world through its practice of appropriating bits and pieces of mainstream culture and converting them into instruments of gay or *queer* signification.

At another time he will speak of "cultural subversion", "appropriation and reinterpretation", and so on. I understand that something similar, although different, does the Deleuze-Guattari machine, for example, with the schizo and schizophrenia, or desire and subjectivation, or the body. Machine effects:

> It works everywhere, either non-stop or dis-continuously. It breathes, it warms up, it eats. It shits, it kisses. What a mistake to have said it. Everywhere machines, and not metaphorically: machines of machines, with their couplings, their connections. An organ-machine connects with a source-machine:
>
> The breast is a machine that produces milk, and the mouth is a machine attached to it. The breast is a machine that produces milk, and the mouth, a machine coupled to it. The mouth of the anorexic vacillates between an eating machine, an anal machine, a talking machine, a breathing machine (asthma crisis). In this way, all "bricoleurs", each one with his own little machines. An organ-machine for an energy machine, always flows and cuts. President Schreber has the rays of heaven in his ass. Solar anus. Moreover, we can be sure that it works; president Schreber feels something, produces something, and can theorise it. Something is produced: machine effects, but not metaphors.
>
> (Deleuze and Guattari, 2002)

There is a "shiny, black truth that lies in delirium", say the authors, and thus open the door to other hetero-topical locations of truth, or at least some of it. Perhaps queer is a field that houses some truth that overflows it and affects us, whether we want it to or not, whether we know it or not.

If schizophrenia "is the universe of the producing and reproducing desiring machines, the universal primary production as the "essential reality of man and nature" (Deleuze and Guattari, 1972), then a thousand and one ways of taking on a body, multiple sexes, and no gender open up.[19]

If "the desiring machines only work by breaking down, breaking down incessantly", we know something of that, those of us who surrender ourselves to formless and unnamed pleasures, that is to say, not nominated by the common denominator of the Name of the father, father of all names.

> And if the perverse one is the one who takes the artifice to the word: speak: you want, you will have, territorialities infinitely more artificial than those that society proposes to us, new families that are completely artificial, secret and lunar societies.
>
> (Deleuze and Guattari, 2002)

The Queer Becoming or the Queerness of Becoming

It will not about producing new crystallizations or a coagulation of identities.

> Becoming is not a correspondence of relationships. But neither is it a resemblance, an imitation.

Let us make artifice the only truth, as Wilde and Genet, García Lorca, and so many others did.

Truth has the structure of artifice

If desiring production is *anedipal*, as Deleuze and Guattari call it in *Anti-Oedipus*, let us blow the lid off the Oedipus, as Melanie Klein could have done and did not, or as Lacan perhaps tried to do and some of his disciples took it upon themselves to remaster it.

The Deleuze-Guattari machine anticipates or prefigures multiple becomings, including in the field of discourses. I would go so far as to say that Donna Haraway, Bruno Latour, and Isabelle Stengers are not without this machine. Thus, it is already proclaimed in *A Thousand Plateaus*:

> a circulation of impersonal affects, an alternative current, which disrupts both signifying projects and subjective feelings, and constitutes a non-human sexuality, – an irresistible deterritorialisation, which annuls in advance the attempts at oedipal, conjugal or professional reterritorialisation (would there be oedipal animals, with which one can "do Oedipus", make a family, my little dog, my kitten, and then other animals which, on the contrary, would drag us into an irresistible devenirnir?
>
> (Deleuze and Guattari [1980] 2002)

Symbiogenesis, multiple entanglements, actants, antispeciesism, posthumanism could be effects of this seventies machine that queers already regard with some suspicion.

> Ultimately, an identification. The whole structuralist critique of the series seems inevitable. To become is neither to progress nor to return according to a series. And, above all, becoming does not occur in the imagination, even when it reaches the cosmic or dynamic level. Animal becomings are not dreams or phantoms. They are perfectly real. But what reality would that be? For if becoming an animal does not consist in becoming the animal or in imitating it, it is also clear that man does not "really" become an animal, just as the animal does not really become something else. Becoming does not produce anything other than itself. It is a false alternative that makes us say: either one imitates or one is.

> What is real is becoming itself, the block of becoming, and not the supposedly fixed terms into which the becoming would transform itself
>
> (Deleuze and Guattari)

Queer, then, as becoming, as a means – medium – and not as an end. A means that makes lives livable that in principle are not. Unproductive and desiring lives.

Body without organs, fluid and slippery, uncreated body[20]

Could it be that *The Man of Wolves* was in search of his own nothingness? The authors of *A Thousand Plateaus* suggest so: was Juanito seeking to become a horse? It would seem so if we read, in addition to *A Thousand Plateaus*, Alberto Carvajal's (2021) extremely scientific text "El performance de las sexualidades" (The performance of sexualities). Schreber hoped to become the woman of God?

If "there are no other drives than one's own agency", then Foucault's Herculine Barbin, or the Agnés of Paul B. Preciado's *The Invention of Gender or the Technocordero who devours wolves* Preciado (2009) differ only in the agency they are capable of. Of course, that's what their lives depend on . . .

Of queerising lx sujetx

> Of a strange subject, without a fixed identity, who wanders on the body without organs, always next to the desiring machines, defined by the part he takes in the product, who gathers everywhere the premium of a becoming or of an avatar, who is born of the states he consumes and is reborn in each state.
>
> (Deleuze and Guattari, 1998)

And what about the social bond, what about the common, and what about the political subject?

Preciado (2014b) echoes Guattari who echoes Deleuze who echoes Paul Klee and speaks of "The missing people". The queer, rather than a people, seems to me more like a deformed, formless monstrosity – a multitude, detached from all affiliation.

Some of this was also anticipated by this fabulous machine Deleuze-Guattari:

> A multiplicity without the unity of an ancestor? It is very simple and everyone knows it, even if it is only talked about in secret. We oppose epidemy to filiation, contagion to inheritance, population by contagion to sexual reproduction, to sexual production. Gangs, human and animal, proliferate with contagions, epidemics, battlefields and catastrophes. It happens as with sterile, sterile children, born of a sexual union that will not reproduce, but which starts again each time, always gaining the same amount of ground. The participations, the unnatural marriages, are the true Nature that runs through the kingdoms. Propagation by

epidemics, by contagion, has nothing to do with the with filiation by inheritance, even if the two subjects mix and have need of each other. The vampire does not filiate, he infects. The difference is that contagion, the epidemic, brings into play completely heterogeneous terms: for example, a man, an animal and a bacterium, a virus, a molecule, a micro-organism. Or, as in the case of the truffle, a tree, a fly and a pig. Combinations that are neither genetic nor structural, inter-kingdom, participations against nature, that is how Nature proceeds, against itself. We are far from filial production, from hereditary reproduction, which only retain as differences a simple duality of sexes within the same species, and small modifications throughout the generations. For us, on the contrary, there are as many sexes as there are terms in symbiosis, as many differences as there are elements involved in a process of contagion. . . . The Universe does not function by filiation.

(Deleuze and Guattari, 2002)

Gilles Deleuze and Felix Guattari, as Leonor Silvestri (2020) rightly says, are white European heterosexual men, but I believe that the most queer thing about their act was precisely to become a machine, to allow me the neologism that is still affecting us.

From the mud of a river: Impasses and assumptions

> Life is something that goes – as we say in French – *à la dérive*. Life runs downstream, touching a bank from time to time, stranding for a moment here and there without anything being understood – and this is the principle of analysis, that nobody understands anything that happens.
>
> (J. Lacan, *On the structure as an immixion of otherness* . . .)

Warning: the writing strategy of this text seems to be that of an interminable digression. Perhaps it is.

i. Diversions to the father[21]

When I was halfway through my analysis, more than ten years after it had begun, we reached an impasse. It wasn't moving. Closer to IPA psychoanalysis at the time, I attributed that impasse to some resistance in me, of course. However, the analytic literature of the time spoke of a resistential analyst-analyst compliance.[22] Then, almost like in the Chapulin colorado, the Mexican TV series by Roberto Gómez Bolaños, I asked myself: and now who will be able to help me?[23]

My analysis took place three times a week at seven o'clock in the morning, so I had to wake up very early each time, and I would go with a different version of the same thing. Fresh dreams – the association with the man with fresh brains[24] is no mere coincidence – which at the time seemed a good sign. However, the impasse also included the dreams; I had not remembered them for a long time, so the sessions passed almost in absolute silence.

One of those days, I woke up with the memory of a dream from that night, just a scene: me as a teenager entering a lonely, cool river, full stop. The associations led us to the Rio Negro, the river on the banks of which I had spent my childhood in a city in the interior of my country. The analyst, in an unusual act for her, does not wait for my associations, she seems to wake up from a long sleep and says something like: "the mud . . . from the river . . . on your feet . . . when you enter the river . . . I have never talked about that".

I am surprised, but something in me unleashes – never better said – a long chain of associations and memories that I thought were lost, of a sensory nature, almost unspeakable, just babbleable. And the analysis, like the water of the river, flows again, vertiginous and alive, very much alive.

After I finished my analysis, I found out that my analyst had spent long periods of time in that same city where I lived and had bathed in that river many times. So I knew – without knowing it – about the mud of the river.

Years later, already on Lacanian shores, the memory of this crucial moment of my analysis comes back to me, and in that practice so habitual in me – which has its origin, it is imposed on me, in puberty – of repeating words and phrases, making them sound over and over again, as if I wanted to squeeze them, to make them exude all their polysemic juice, I repeat: mud from the river, mud from the river . . . barrio, Barrios . . . my paternal surname!

My father was called Negro, Negro Barrios – Río Negro, mud from the Rio Negro . . .[25]

Then other associations become unavoidable for me. In my artistic practice in the visual arts, but also in poetry, I soon feel the need to localise what I do, and it seems strange to me, a bit kitsch, camp, baroque, neo-baroque,. . .

I call one of my works: muddy chimerical hydra . . . The mud insists.

Versions of the father, perversions, but of which father? The father does not exist. He is made to exist.

There are fathers. There was my father.

My parents belonged to very different social classes; my mother the daughter of a once prosperous merchant, my father the son of a nurse – all father, mother, sister. The class struggle, embraced by both from different versions of a guerrilla left, not just political – even if they remained more at the level of support groups – ran through my family without that being said.[26] The meeting of the two branches of the family was always an uncomfortable tension and we – my parents, my siblings and I – in the midst of it, tried to "have a peaceful party", although clearly we did not always succeed.

My father would sometimes retaliate – shaking off his subalternity – when my mother and some of us would get very theoretical, very know-it-all, telling us that we were suffering from "enlightened despotism". This syntagma will insist on me, whenever I or some others seem to embody this subjective and political position in the field of psychoanalysis, though not only there.

ii. *My mother was not a crocodile*[27]

And it didn't take a stick in her mouth to stop her from eating us.

The mother doesn't exist, my mother exists

Can we continue to maintain with Lacan (1992) that:

> The role of the mother is the desire of the mother. This is capital. The desire of the mother is not something that can be endured as it is, that can be indifferent to them. It always wreaks havoc. It is being inside the mouth of a crocodile, that is the mother. You don't know which fly might bite her and suddenly she goes and closes her mouth. That is the mother's desire?

What does it always mean in psychoanalysis, is there a universal? The mother does not exist.

My mother, a feminist of difference, did not seek to complete herself with her children, much less phallically. And there were many occasions when we noticed that her desire was caused by other objects. I looked to my grandmother and my paternal aunt for those crocodiles who wanted to devour me while I kept escaping from their mouths.

In that city, on the banks of a black river, I heard about Lacan as a child. A philosophy teacher, recently arrived from Paris, was practising psychoanalysis with her students. One of those students was my mother. In my memory, which I am sure will be a cover-up – I wonder if any of them are not – this analyst told me that Lacan dressed in a black cloak[28] (another insistence, that of black) and said that he was psychotic. He struck me as a wise magician figure, who not only was not afraid of madness, but who embraced it and challenged his audience not to pretend any normality.

For years I forgot all this. I entered the Freudian path, a less frightening father who would open the doors of psychoanalysis and probably of social inclusion, of the hetero-oedipal, white, bourgeois, normal. Until – near the end of my analysis – a sort of wave, or rather, one of those whirlpools of a river that, according to the legends of my people, could suck you in and drown you – the river has no arms, it was said – burst in session after session, and Lacan as a signifier came to function as a magnet,[29] a master signifier, of a thousand and one significations. In the end, my analyst – I suppose she was also a bit fed up with it – said: "Well, go to the Lacanians if you want to!

The Lacanians don't exist. . . . She didn't know it, and neither did I, yet.

iii. *Of getting muddy, of the unconscious as politics, and of the politics of the unconscious*

You may ask yourselves, what is the point of all this personal history, and who cares, you may even think. However, if the personal is political – as the feminists of the seventies taught us – I propose two other enunciations: *the singular is political* and there is a *politics of the singular*.

There is a psychoanalysis that pretends to make the symptom its politics, and seems to see there the most singular aspect of its operation. However, Freud and Lacan were already able to see – or at least mention – the political dimension of the symptom – with regard to Dora, for example – although perhaps we have not yet been able to draw all its consequences from this.[30]

Freud assenting to Dora's truth about the family entanglement to which she is made the object, although taking responsibility for her part in it. Subjective responsibility, Miller et al. will say.[31] Lacan (1984b) – somewhat more cautious, though not too much so – in *Intervention on the transference* will point out:

> Dora entered the illness, dragging the whole world to recognise her as ill – which ironically responds to her refusal to continue her supporting function for their common ailment (not all the benefits of neurosis are for the exclusive benefit of the neurotic).

This is what I call the *political function of neurosis*. There is a psychoanalysis that seeks to establish clear boundaries and to establish the political function of neurosis. It is Lacan who never tires of enunciating: this is not psychoanalysis![32]; threatened in his patrimony and at most granting himself a gracious licence a la Miller (2021): to make himself docile to the trans, as Lacan in *Television* will say of Freud: docile to hysteria. *Our Master plays the slave*, as Patricio Rey and Los redonditos de ricota would say.[33] But the Master does not give up his place so easily, as we know.

Fortunately, or by necessity, there is also another psychoanalysis that renounces all pretensions of domination, all colonial dreams of purity and calls itself hybrid, as in Thamy Ayouch's *Psychoanalysis and Hybridity* (2020), or as I propose in this book: *Degenerating psychoanalysis*. I prefer not to adjectivise psychoanalysis, but rather to make it suffer the effects of an accursed verb that alludes to being out of gender, impure, abnormal, aberrant.

It is not about a "war of ideas", as The Son-in-law – or The Godfather – will say, but about what we are willing to accept, which lives, which erotics, which sufferings? And which not. And of how much we are prepared to put into crisis, without catastrophism: "change everything so that nothing changes", or economic or political calculation *aggiornamientos*.

The Master sees only two possibilities: to become docile or to dominate. Psychoanalysis does not exist.

Someone, a Frenchman, said in the school of psychoanalysis of which I am a member that "there is no psychoanalysis in Spanish". It was a provocation, of course. Many were offended, but I was not. It seemed to me an interesting challenge that I decided to take up: perhaps he is right, as long as we do not do in our language, even in our language, what Lacan did in his language with Freud's psychoanalysis in German.

If, as Lacan (1984a) says in passing in *L'etourdit*, psychoanalysis is *a practice of saying*, this implies not sparing ourselves from giving an account of what language does to us in an analysis. And the saying of these effects of saying-writing – all together – perhaps provides the conditions of possibility for psychoanalysis in Spanish.

That is why I have been saying for some time now that I write texts-performance, monster texts, half-spoken, derivative, proliferating, muddy and slippery, associative and dissociative, hollowed out, incomplete, even impossible.

I thought of making a list of questions I would have liked to ask Jacques Lacan, had I known him. Today I am asking them to you. The idea of a list made me uneasy, so I decided to continue asking questions indirectly, camouflaged in lucubrations, affirmations, and comments, only apparently rhetorical. Many times, reading Freud and/or Lacan, I have thought that much of what they seem to affirm are nothing more than questions that are never asked, never formulated as such. Descriptions of things they observe in their practice from previous readings.

First came reading; in theory, of course, not in the subjective constitution, there first came writing. Then it will be a saying that in the best of cases will have the effect of writing due to the operation of the interventions of the person who occupies the analyst function there. It is precisely for this reason that the readings we make read us. And the ones we don't make?

The unconscious is politics, Miller reminds us, but which unconscious is it? There is a politics of the apolitical, ahistorical, non-located unconscious. There is a psychoanalysis that reads this Lacanian sentence as "there is no politics of psychoanalysis other than the unconscious", that is to say: the unconscious is unaware of politics or knows no politics other than its own.

However, it is repeated: The unconscious is the discourse of the Other, Desire is the desire of the Other, which Other is it about? The Other does not exist . . . and yet it produces effects. Does anyone believe that the symbolic order is immutable? Do patriarchy, heteronormativity as a political regime, capitalism constitute the symbolic order or not?[34] If so, what is the politics of an unconscious that is politics? Of course, it is not a question of doing politics in analysis, but perhaps of *a particular doing with the political of a singular saying*. That is my wager.

Someone says something about the DSM in session. I hear – all together – "wish me". That is all. It may not sound like much; however, I can't help but notice the political subversion of this intervention that reads "I'm sorry". The desire of the individual is a word that says of his desire, hiding itself in a medical, psychiatric saying.

An intervention that I consider to be the opposite, made from a different politics of the unconscious – if you will pardon the parricidal gesture – will be Lacan's intervention with a Jewish analysand. Many psychoanalysts never cease to admire this intervention of Lacan's recounted by Suzanne Hommel, following a dream in relation to the Gestapo and the persecution of Jews. Lacan transforms Gestapo into "geste a peu", a caress on the analysand's face. A commentator says: "the Gestapo will no longer be the Gestapo" from this gesture of Lacan's. It seems to me a lot, certainly too much. It smacks of reparation and the reduction of horror to a demand for love. It smacks of a depoliticisation, very political indeed, of a reality that is imagined from a political symbolism that is too political. The fact that it is a testimony does not oblige us to assent "meekly" to its reading, I will say, not without irony.

Who can bear witness to oneself without opacity? And when it is a question of transference, what is one testifying about? Even less so when this testimony is collected by Gerard Miller – in case any other specimen of familiarism was needed – in a hagiographic documentary, the genius of Jacques Lacan.[35] There is still a lot of mud to get muddy with, anal jouissance one might say, analysis of one jouissance or another – in the plural – multiple jouissances, in flight, *devenires monstrxs*.

Two years ago, I installed a work in an exhibition centre in Montevideo, a work I called *Artista de mierda* – in a nod to the work Mierda de artista by Piero Manzoni –[36] and I brought real shit into a museum. The centre's management feared that it would smell bad, but given that the work had been shortlisted for a major prize in the visual arts, they could only agree to its installation. The faeces of dozens of artists could be contemplated in a showcase that was a Greek present[37] to art and its claim to the sublime. Today I'm tempted to rename this book: *Analista de mierda*, because that's what it's also about, about becoming deject.

Psychoanalysis of the end or the end of psychoanalysis?

The future of a disillusionment

> I will mitigate my ardor and admit the possibility that I too am pursuing an illusion.
> —Sigmund Freud, *The Coming of an Illusion* (1988b)

i.

Does psychoanalysis still have something to say today? I don't think so. This is not obvious, even though I have been practising it for thirty-three years.

For a long time it was believed that psychoanalysts – said in the masculine, in an attempt to pass it off as a universal – knew something. And as Lacan said in Louvain in 1972: "the last straw is that they themselves believed it". For many years, psychoanalysis operated as a privileged matrix of subjectivation in the West and as a hegemonic matrix of sexuation. Likewise, for many years psychoanalysis contributed, explicitly or not, to a conception of "the human".

Psychoanalysis is not humanism, we say. But is it enough to state this for it to cease to be so? In recent decades, multiple warnings have questioned – when they have not openly refuted – some of this supposed knowledge: feminisms, queer theory, decolonial warnings, antispeciesism, etc. Authors such as Deleuze and Guattari, Donna Haraway, Bruno Latour, Isabelle Stengers, Viveiros de Castro, and Deborah Danowski, among many others, take approaches that, from various biases, place psychoanalysis more in a position of learning than of supposed mastery or domination of some knowledge.

Monique Wittig pointing out heterosexuality as a political regime, Gayle-Rubin making the sex-gender system visible, Judith Butler warning about the performative character of gender and also of sex, Paul B. Preciado questioning the regime of sexual difference as a political epistemology, the basis of a scientific religion, Oyeronki Oyewumi making transparent the invention of women as an invention of the West, and much earlier Karen Horney discussing penis envy, and so many others, make any supposedly psychoanalytic certainty impossible.

ii.

For some time now, we have been living through a climatic and ecological collapse that is devastating the earth. Global warming and its multiple effects make visible the passage of humanity from a biological agent to a geological force. The Anthropocene is the name of the disaster of which humanity is the main agent.

The nature-culture distinction no longer holds. There is a multiplicity of beings and objects with agency, actants – capable of affecting and being affected – producing effects. Everything that produces effects exists. There is "a tremor in being" that, according to Timothy Morton (2018) and others, enables other non-correlationist ontologies, object-oriented ontologies, ontologies without a subject. Hyperobjects that relate in an other, non-human temporality. "The world is ceasing to be Kantian".[38] God, the Soul, and the World, the three Kantian transcendental ideas are dying out. The world is the last metaphysical remnant, almost a fossil, one might say. Gaia bursts forth in a thousand and one ways. Gaia is not the Earth.

Isabelle Stengers (2017) says: "To name Gaia as "the intruder" is also to characterise her as blind, in the manner of everything that intrudes, to the destruction she causes. The response to be created is not a "response to Gaia" but a response both to what provoked her intrusion and to the consequences of that intrusion". Gaia acknowledges her trauma and erupts in many ways, reminding us that we so-called *humans* are not the only beings capable of agency. Abiotic beings make pandemics. Humanism shows its exhaustion as a speciesist, patriarchal, colonial, and modern paradigm. Multispecies alliances, hybridisations, mutations, sympoiesis, and cyborg agency open up other possibilities of existence for all.

Juliana Fausto (2017), in *Cosmopolitics of Animals*, warns that it is necessary to explore the place of *animals other than humans* – as she calls them – in the polis, to liberate them from human politics that do not consider them capable of agency. Donna Haraway (2019b) invites us, or perhaps it would be better to say urges us, to produce other narratives for life on a wounded planet.

We inhabit tentacular, rhizomatic, heterarchical, fluid, inconsistent, proliferating drifting worlds. Our lives take place in dissipative systems, the probabilistic never excludes chance.

We inhabit spectral worlds.

Some time ago, with a foot in Jacques Derrida's text (1995), *Expectros de Marx. The state of debt, the work of mourning and the new international, as* well as with the works of Mark Fisher (2018) and others, the spectral has put the dead/living dichotomy in tension, and various authors have unfolded the consequences of this problematisation of a metaphysics of presence, which makes possible, among other things, a way out of the "humanist treatment of otherness", as Gabriela Balcarce (2016–2017) and others point out.

In our countries, moreover, having suffered dictatorships, with torture and disappearances, as well as indigenous exterminations and the slave trade, the spectral acquires an unusual political potency while pointing to an ever-open colonial wound. If we add to this the existence of other, non-Catholic spiritualities, for which coexistence with spirits is part of the everyday life of the people, the spectral – once the spiritual – ritual coloniality, a far from minor effect and method of conquest-colonisation, has been noted – increases its vital consequences.

Surely someone is asking: how does this affect psychoanalysis? So, as they say, as if a button were enough, I will only say that, for example, this other consideration of presence could enable a critical revisiting of the notion of the *Umheimlich*, the ominous, so dear to a certain psychoanalysis. Or of the *fort da*, or of the symbolic, or of the three registers: real-symbolic-imaginary, and of course, of mourning, which seems to me to be no small thing. On this occasion, I can only mention this as a point to be deployed at another time.

iii.

As a discourse of the real – in the Lacanian sense – psychoanalysis inhabits a world where multiple discourses about the real proliferate. Nothing assures its privilege with respect to any truth.

Freud lived through a time of civilisational mutation; the decimononic culture had to make room for a growing techno-scientific acceleration as well as an intensification of the production of consumer goods, the appearance of the theory of relativity, the production of antibiotics, advances in molecular biology, DNA, etc., which increased confidence – in order not to lose the opportunity to be provocative, we would say faith – in progress and in reason, fundamentally in scientific reason.

For Freud, the illusion – the enemy of reason – is religion. For us, on the other hand, the disillusionment is with modernity, humanity and humanism. Gloria Leff (2021) recently published her book *Lo oculto, verdad indómita. Freud, István Hollos . . . and others*, where – among other virtues of the book – it is clear that the so-called "occult" was and is an issue that is not alien to psychoanalysis.

Modernity – as we know today – is the illusion: a colonial, civilising, racist, speciesist illusion, and a long purpose.

Says Freud:

> If you have lived for a long time within a given culture and have therefore often endeavoured to explore its origins and developmental path, you will at some point be tempted to look in the other direction and wonder about the distant destiny that awaits that culture and the changes it is destined to undergo. But he will soon realise that there are several factors that make such an enquiry worthless

> in advance. First of all, because there are very few people who are capable of comprehending the whole fabric of human affairs in all its ramifications. For most people it has become necessary to confine themselves to one field or to a few; and yet the less one knows about the past and the present, the more uncertain one's judgement of the future will be. Secondly, because it is precisely in such a judgement that the subjective expectations of the individual play a part which is to be considered considerable; and these, in turn, are dependent on purely personal factors, such as his own experience, his more or less special attitude towards life as prescribed by his temperament, his success or his failure. Finally, there is the astonishing fact that human beings generally experience their present as *naïve*, without being able to appreciate its contents; they should first distance themselves from it, i.e., the present has to become the past if they are to gain from it.
>
> (1988)

Naivete with respect to the present, says Freud; negationism, says Deborah Danowski (2019), which no longer includes individual death, unthinkable for Freud, but the imminent possibility of the disappearance of humanity, even of planet earth. Global warming, planetary crisis, climate change become almost euphemisms to avoid talking about the end. The end of the world that never ceases to produce versions.

"For most people it has become necessary to confine themselves to a single field or to a few", says Freud, at the antipodes of the epistemic-cosmogonic point of view that is essential today. As Bruno Latour (2007) characterises it, we live in skeins, we are hybrids, back in the Gordian knot that symbiotises knowledge and knowledges, always in translation, always in a network.

In this sense, it is necessary to recover the notion of cosmogonies, of the creation of worlds, of cosmopolitanism. Specific knowledge is nothing but epistemic drift.

Psychoanalysis gave discourse to "the human", from a position of species exceptionalism, which today we would call speciesist. Let us see how Freud puts it in this text: "Human culture – I mean everything in which human life has risen above its animal conditions and is distinguished from animal life" (Latour, 2007).

And he adds:

> encompasses all the knowledge and know-how that people have acquired in order to govern the forces of nature and to extract from it goods that satisfy their needs; on the other hand, it comprises all the rules necessary to regulate the reciprocal links between people and, in particular, the distribution of affordable goods.
>
> (Latour, 2007)

The human – let me continue to use the masculine, since man is obviously the model of the human – is outside nature and governs it. Relay the biblical injunction: "Be fruitful, multiply, fill the earth and subdue it; have dominion over the fish of the sea, over the birds of the air, over the living creatures that move upon the earth" (Genesis 1:28).

Let's look at a few more pearls:

> If in the beginning it was thought that what was essential in it was the subjugation of nature in order to obtain the means of life, and that it was possible to avert the dangers threatening it by the appropriate distribution of the latter among people, now the centre of gravity seems to have shifted from the material to the mental. The decisive factor will be whether (and to what extent) it is possible to alleviate the burden that the sacrifice of the drives imposes on men, to reconcile them with what is still necessary and to compensate them for it.
>
> (Freud)

The human being as a being of culture pays for his exceptionalism with sexual and aggressive drives. It is no longer a question of satisfying his "animal" material needs, but of renouncing the satisfaction of his libidinal and aggressive desires. Perhaps the political consequences of these renunciations have not been sufficiently pointed out.

But let Freud speak:

> Just as indispensable as the compulsion to cultural work is *the rule of the masses by a minority, for the masses are indolent and unintelligent, they do not love the renunciation of the drives, it is impossible to convince them of their inevitability by argument, and their individuals corroborate each other in their tolerance of their debauchery*. Only through the influence of archetypal individuals whom the masses accept as their leaders is it possible to move them to the work and abstinence that the survival of culture requires. All is well if these leaders are people who have a superior vision of the objective necessities of life and who have risen to the level of control of the masses.
>
> But, in their eagerness not to lose their influence, they are exposed to the risk of making more concessions to the masses than the masses make to them, and therefore it seems necessary for them to have the means of power to remain independent of the masses.
>
> (Latour, 2007) (Emphasis added)

In other words, the government of the masses presupposes the promotion to power of "archetypal" leaders – how strange this term sounds in Freud's mouth, a Freud we might call Jungian just for the pleasure of annoying him post mortem. A whole political programme, of government . . . Then it will be said that psychoanalysis is not political. Civilisation and barbarism seems to be the sub-text or the unwritten intertext, and therefore the most effective.[39]

Freud, however, seems to be aware that modernity as "the great cultural experiment now taking place in the vast country between Europe and Asia" is in trouble and seems to anticipate Stengers' Gaia:

> But no man falls into the delusion that nature is already conquered; and few dare to hope that man will ever completely subdue it. There are the elements, which seem to mock every human yoke: The earth, which trembles and tears apart, abyssing everything human and every work of man; the water, which rages and drowns everything; the typhoon, which sweeps away everything in its path; the diseases, which we have not long ago discerned as the attacks of other living beings; finally, the painful enigma of death, for which no balm has so far been found, nor is it likely to be discovered. With these violences nature rises up against us, grandiose, cruel, merciless; thus she again brings before our eyes our feebleness and weakness.

HOW TO RESIST THE COMING BARBARISM?

> We thought we had been saved by the work of culture. One of the few joyful and comforting impressions one can have of humanity is when, in the face of a catastrophe unleashed by the elements, it forgets its cultural routine, all its difficulties and internal enmities, and remembers the great common task: to preserve itself against the unequal power of nature.
>
> (Freud)

Like many things in Freud – and also in Lacan – one does not know whether one is confronted with a description of the present state of things – not without a certain pessimism or essentialist fatalism – or with a justification of the *status quo*.

Thus, for example, in the face of the oppressed classes:

> As far as the restrictions affecting certain classes of society are concerned, we are confronted with very visible constellations, which have never been unknown. It is to be expected that these relegated classes will envy the privileged their prerogatives and will do everything to get rid of their "plus" of deprivation. Where this is not possible, a certain degree of permanent discontent will be consolidated within that culture, which can lead to dangerous rebellions. But if a culture has not been able to avoid the fact that the satisfaction of a certain number of its members is premised on the oppression of others, perhaps the majority (and this is the case in all present-day cultures), it is understandable that the oppressed develop an intense hostility towards that culture which they make possible through their work, but of whose goods they share only to a very limited extent. They are therefore not expected to internalise cultural prohibitions; on the contrary, they are unwilling to recognise them, they strive to destroy culture itself, and possibly even to cancel its rewards. The hostility of these classes to culture is so manifest that the more latent hostility of the better-off strata of society has been overlooked.
>
> (Freud)

And here comes the sentence by which we are reconciled, at least momentarily, with Freud:

> It goes without saying that a culture that leaves such a large number of its members dissatisfied and pushes them to revolt has no prospect of lasting preservation, nor does it deserve it.

The same is true of the anthropomorphisation of the non-human: "it is connatural for human beings to personify everything they try to conceive in order to govern it afterwards".

With the added bonus – a point in Freud's favour – that here the interpretation of the phenomenon includes a dimension of power, which could well satisfy Foucault and his bid to unveil the social relations of power that constitute the microphysics of every social bond. Let's conclude for today with Freud's demarcation of the term *illusion* in this text, which enables interesting drifts outside of all naive realism, not without political consequences that touch on the conquest of America as well as Nazism:

> . . . *illusions*, I have to clarify the meaning of the term. An illusion is not the same as an error; nor is it necessarily an error. Aristotle's opinion that the vermin bred in filth, which is still held by ignorant people today, was an error, as was that of the physicians of an earlier generation that *tabes dorsalis* was the result of sexual excesses. It would be unwise to call these errors illusions. On the other hand, it was Columbus' illusion that he had discovered a new sea route to the Indies. The participation of his desire in this error is more than evident. The thesis of certain nationalists that the Indo-Germans are the only race fit for culture can be described as an illusion, as can the belief – only destroyed by psychoanalysis – that the child lacks sexuality. The characteristic feature of the delusion is that it always derives from human desires; in this respect it is close to the delusional idea of psychiatry, although it is not identified with it either, even if we dispense with the complex edifice of the delusional idea. The essential feature of the latter is its contradiction with actual reality; on the other hand, the non-necessary delusion – the delusion of the human being – is not necessarily the same as the delirium of psychiatry. The mind is false, that is to say, unrealistic or contradictory to reality.
>
> (Freud)

It would be interesting today to put this illusion/reality dichotomy in tension with two contemporary notions such as Nick Land's Hyperstition and Timothy Morton's Hyperobjects. Hyperstition as fiction that creates the future it predicts and hyperobjects as viscous, non-locatable entities, on a scale much larger than the human scale, which makes Morton say: "the present is nowhere, the objects are never present".

To conclude, Freud opens the umbrella before it rains. In other words, he foresees the criticisms of his text and defends himself:

> And if I now come to the fore with such disgusting manifestations, there will be those who will be more than willing to move from me to psychoanalysis. Now you can see, they will say, where psychoanalysis leads. The mask has fallen: to disown God and the ethical ideal, as we had always suspected. To prevent us from discovering this, we were cajoled that psychoanalysis does not possess a worldview, nor could it create one.
>
> (Freud)

Interestingly, the notion of cosmos returns here as a worldview, but Freud seeks to dissociate himself from it:

> Criticism has undermined the evidential force of religious documents; natural science has investigated the errors they contain, and comparative study has recorded the striking and fatal resemblance between the religious representations we revere and the spiritual productions of primitive peoples and ages. The scientific spirit engenders a determined attitude towards the things of this world; in matters of religion it pauses for a moment, hesitates, and finally crosses the threshold here too. The more accessible the treasures of our knowledge become to human beings, the more widespread is the renunciation of religious faith, at first only of its antiquated and shocking garments, but later also of its fundamental premises.

Freud's scientific illusion is underpinned by the refusal of religion understood as abandonment of the parental home – father and God (Catholic, it should be noted, although Freud extends this to all ideas of God) are one and the same thing in Freud's assertion:

> And now we are entitled to say that it is probably high time to replace, as in the analytic treatment of the neurotic, the results of repression by those of intellectual work in accordance with the *ratio*. . . . Evidently, man will thus find himself in a difficult situation: he will have to confess his total worthlessness, his insignificance in the fabric of the universe; he will cease to be the centre of creation, the object of the tender care of a kind Providence. He will find himself in the same situation as the child who has left the parental home in which so much warmth and comfort reigned. But is it not true that infantilism is destined to be overcome? Man cannot remain a child in himself; in the end he has to throw himself out into the world. This can be called "education for reality"; need I reveal to you, still, that the sole purpose of my writing is to draw attention to the necessity of this progress?

Almost a hundred years later, the parental home to be abandoned seems to have been extended or shifted from the Freudian axis. Perhaps it is the earth itself and humanity, exceptionalism and the subject, heteronormativity and capacitism, racism, reason, and patriarchy, that are to be abandoned.

The future of disillusionment.

Heterosexuality of love: In praise of a certain illegibility or the invention of other ways of affecting oneself

Can love not be heterosexual? What would a non-heterosexual love be? I start from the hypothesis that romantic love is a *dispositive*, that is to say, in the sense that it is a *dispositive in* the Foucauldian sense of the term:

> a resolutely heterogeneous ensemble comprising discourses, institutions, architectonic habilitations, regulatory decisions, laws, administrative measures, scientific statements, philosophical, moral and philanthropic propositions. In short, between the said and the unsaid, these are the elements of the device. The dispositif itself is the network that we weave between these elements. . . . By dispositif I mean a kind of formation which, at a given moment, has had as its main function to respond to an urgency.
>
> (Foucault, 1994)

And if we continue with the quotation:

> Thus, the dispositif is always inscribed in a play of power, but also linked to a limit or limits of knowledge, which give birth to it but, above all, condition it. This is the dispositif: strategies of power relations sustaining types of knowledge, and sustained by them.
>
> (Foucault, 1994)

For Foucault, devices produce what they were created for. That is why it is not possible to reappropriate them. An insult can be reappropriated, but not a device. A little before Javier Saez said and wrote it, I had been thinking and sharing with some colleagues from the school of psychoanalysis to which I belong, my suspicions about love.

It was in this way that Saez's text (2015) *El amor es heterosexual (Love is heterosexual)* only confirmed that he was not so far wrong. After a porn punk feminist meeting in Donosti, organised by (at the time Beatriz) Preciado, Saez noticed a generalised celebration of love that caught her attention and made her think:

> . . . if the rhetoric of love is just another discourse and another practice that we have adopted from the heterosexual regime. In any case, it is a totally harmless and domesticated discourse, something that does not bother the patriarchal and homophobic system at all. On the contrary, buns, queers and even transgender people are much better digested and accepted when they have a father ("what healthy boys, they are no longer promiscuous") and above all

> when they proclaim "their love" ("look how nice they are, they love each other; they are just like us"). As Foucault said, what bothers power is not homosexual relations, but friendship. That is to say, the possibility of creating networks of friends, support, affection, solidarity, which are difficult to locate, which escape social control and go beyond the binary individualist or liberal model: "couple-love-marriage".
>
> (Saez, 2015)

I do not think it is by chance that in this quotation Foucault speaks first of "affection, tenderness, friendship, fidelity, camaraderie, companionship" and only later of "*s'aimer*", which I translate as "to love each other, not to be loved", and which he characterises as: relationships of multiple intensities, of variable colours, of imperceptible movements, of changing forms. Even in *On Friendship as a Way of Life*, Foucault (1981) does not seem to need love to cover the experience of pleasure that unites two men: "They have to invent from A to Z a relationship still without form which is friendship: that is to say the sum of all the things through which one and the other can give pleasure to each other".

I wonder why to equate this other mode of relationship "of changing forms" or even "without form" with the corset or the wardrobe of the signifier love. What we take out of the door comes back in through the window. In decolonial theory, we speak of internal colonialism. Should we speak of internal heteronormativity (with all the co-miles corresponding to "internal")? It is a question, it seems to me, of making room for an asceticism and an invention with respect to the known, already invented and inventoried ways of affecting oneself.

Foucault says:

> Asceticism as the renunciation of pleasure has a bad reputation. But askesis is something else. It is the work that one does on oneself in order to transform oneself or to make appear that self that happily is never attained. Is this not our problem today? Asceticism has been given a holiday. It is up to us to advance on a homosexual asceticism that would make us work on ourselves and invent, I don't say discover, a way of being that is still improbable.

Saez seemed to summon the underworld, and all or almost all his comrades in a fissured queer camp threw themselves upon him. He received aggravations and even psychological interpretations of his "love problem".

Preciado would soon rectify his position radically:

> I would like to celebrate 14 February by confessing a secret to you. Let's say this will be my Valentine's Day present. This summer I stopped believing in love. In love as a couple. It was not progressive. It was a sharp blow: the order of my thoughts changed and my desire was radically altered. Or perhaps it was the other way round? I discovered myself desiring differently and the ideas fell of their own weight. Although I am an atheist in theology and a nominalist in

> philosophy, love had so far resisted the hermeneutics of suspicion and the harassment of deconstruction. On the side of virtue, the rhetoric of love persisted in me like a neoplatonic remnant of years of meta-physical training.
>
> (Preciado, 2015)

We have a bad memory. Guy Hocquenghem (2009) had already sentenced: "the couple, the most restrictive form of loving and social life that has ever been massively experienced in the history of mankind". Then it was Halperin, in *How to be Gay* (2015), who alerted me to the heterosexuality of a dramaturgy of affects and the existence of another way of being affected, a way that constitutes the queerest of the gay. A way of doing with pain and suffering, and also a renunciation of social empathy and respectability (which we used to call bourgeois).

Thus humour acquires a political-affective function and makes room for another politics of the affections:

> To use one's own grief as a tool of humor, to refuse to exempt oneself from the irony with which one regards all other social identities and personifications of accepted social roles, is, in effect, to level social differences (. . .) not to pretend to be taken seriously and to renounce the right to the empathy of others, to sentimentality.
>
> (Halperin)

Then came my disappointment with Halperin (2019) with his text *Queer Love*, which for me constitutes a step backwards with respect to *How to be Gay. In Queer Love*, Halperin, while acknowledging and quoting Berlant, states:

> Since it is the bond of patriotism and family, love defines governance in its nuclear form, as a mechanism of internal monitoring through which the subject returns to and reproduces desire as a plebiscite on the normal. . . . The installation of romantic love as a fundamental human bond has been central to the normalisation of heterosexuality and femininity in consumer culture; it has become a way of expressing desires and desires for the sexuality of the human being.
>
> It has become a way of expressing desires for a normal life . . ., defining the normativity of the modern self much more than a category such as "sexuality" does.

He proposes to consider queer love as a "counter-conduct":

> Queer love could then be re-established with the status of what Arnold Davidson calls, following Michel Foucault, a "counter-conduct". Once we recover that vitality, that sensitivity to the queerness of lesbian and gay men's love, we can then come to see its expressions as forms of tactical resistance to the standardisation of emotional life in contemporary society.
>
> (Davidson, 2011, in Halperin, 2019)

That is, far from problematising the very notion of love, it produces a deviant variant. Consistent with his idea of queer as *inversions* of the heteronormal world, as operations or practices of deviance – perhaps it would be better to say *practices of the deviant* – he produces his inverted love.

However, personally, I believe that the invertible, the deviable, the reappropriable, has its limits, its points of impossibility. Just as Oedipus does not seem to me invertible, gay-cizable or queerisable, neither does love. Oedipus and romantic love, couple love, are dispositives of sex-affective normalisation, matrices of subjectivation and sexuation, key pieces of the sex-gender system, compulsory heterosexuality and patriarchy. Even reminding us that:

> in fact, the task facing gay men is nothing other than a kind of "homosexual asceticism", as Foucault calls it, "that makes us work on ourselves and invent, I do not say discover [since there is no existing form of life that would serve that purpose], a way of being that is still improbable.
>
> (Foucault, 1981)

Halperin insists on upholding the term *love.*

One of the things that have always seemed to me to be the most revulsive and promising in queerfeminist subversion are the operations in language that it becomes essential to produce, to invent, to assent to its occurrence, since social relations of power permeate a sexual politics of the language that speaks to us, by which we are spoken to.

On the other hand, even today there are those who invoke Greek *paideia* as a demonstration of the viability of another form of "love", the love of boys. Many of them call themselves Foucauldians, or at least readers of Foucault. It never ceases to amaze me.

If we read "The Use of Pleasures", in *History of Sexuality* (Foucault, 1984), it becomes clear that the so-called love of the many is an erotic-political practice of production of future citizens, future rulers of the polis. A polis that is a society of masters and in which the maintenance of power and the supreme value of virility are the flipside of the ghosts of passivity and feminisation of men:

> Loving boys was a "free" practice in the sense that it was not only permitted by law (except in particular circumstances) but also accepted by opinion. Moreover, it found solid support in various institutions (military or pedagogical). It had its religious roots in the rites and festivals in which the divine powers were called upon to protect it. Finally, it was a practice that was culturally valued by a whole literature that praised it and a reflection on its excellence. But all this was mixed with very different attitudes: contempt for young men who were too easy or too interested, disqualification of effeminate men.
>
> (Foucault, 1984)

In many ways, Foucault shows, problematises, the eroticism that makes young men not "objects of pleasure" – that would be inadmissible, given the non-servile, aristocratic character of young men – but "subjects of pleasure", in an adult-youth, lover-beloved game preparatory to the political functions to be assumed in adulthood:

> that the pleasures to be gained from such a relationship required a different moral form from that which was required when it came to loving a woman. In this kind of relationship, the pleasures do not reveal, in the one who experiences them, a strange nature, but their use required a stylistics of its own. It is a fact that, in Greek culture, masculine love was the subject of a whole effervescence of thought, reflection and discussion about the forms it should take or the value it should be given. It would be insufficient to see in this activity of discourse anything other than the immediate and spontaneous translation of a free practice, thus seeking to express itself naturally.
>
> (Foucault, 1984)

And he adds, in case it is not clear:

> To see only in all these precautions taken and in the interest shown in them the proof that this love was free is to miss the essential point, it is to ignore the difference made between this sexual behaviour and the others about which no one was concerned to know how they were to develop.

Rarely has the *political function of an erotic* been more clearly demonstrated. If we still want to call this love, then you will agree with me that it is a political device that makes an erotic its instrument. The same is true of romantic love. If we agree with what Louis George-Tin (2015) describes as the genealogy of heterosexuality in *The Invention of Heterosexual Culture*, we will see that the passage from chivalrous love to courtly love marks the turning point of the invention of heterosexuality as a culture and of its device that generates the conditions of possibility: love:

> One might have to ask whether hetero-sexual cultures, i.e., those in which attraction to the other sex is represented, cultivated and celebrated, are not a particular case which, for historical reasons linked to economic and colonial expansion, have appeared as a general rule.
>
> (Tin 2015)

I find it interesting that this author speaks of "sociosexual dispositif" to refer to heterosexuality as a culture that makes "amorous heterosexuality" more than a practice.

The chivalric culture that preceded heterosexuality was a homoerotic culture, of masculine, virile friendships, of comradeship between men. Duby will call it "virile love", but it is nevertheless an erotics much closer to passionate friendship and homosociality as the basis of an epic, virile society.

Romantic love will come as "absolute love that leads to death" with *Tristan and Isolde* and *Romeo and Juliet*. The same had already been pointed out by Denis de Rougemont (1945) in the now classic *Love and the West*:

> That the chord of *love and death* should be the one that promotes in us the deepest resonances is a fact that already establishes, at first sight, the prodigious success of the *novel*. There are other, more secret reasons for seeing in it a definition of Western consciousness.

Rougemont goes even further, bringing love and adultery almost to the point of equivalence:

> Let us tighten the siege around this contradiction by an effort which *must* seem unpleasant, since it tends to destroy an illusion. To affirm that love-passion means, in fact, adultery, is to insist on the reality that our cult of love both disguises and transfigures; it is to bring to light that which this cult conceals, rejects and refuses to name in order to allow us a burning abandonment to that which we would not dare to claim. The very resistance that the reader will experience in recognising that passion and adultery are often confused in our society is not the first proof of this paradoxical fact: that we want passion and disgrace on condition that we never confess that we want them as such?

Isn't this tragic, dramatic gamble what Halperin calls the "heterosexual gaze" or "dramatic gaze"?

Some time ago, in the field of erotics and discourses that we wrongly call queer – and which I prefer to call the *degeneradx* field – the so-called *affective turn* made its appearance which, together with the so-called anti-social turn, constitute for me today two keys to reading dissident erotics, which *betray* – to put it with the ambiguity that this term has for Jean Genet, which I have already worked on in other texts – cisheteronormativity.

In my text "De los afectos como política de lo subjetivo" (On affects as politics of the subjective), I said:

> As Laurent Berlant, Nicolás Cuello, Mariela Solana, Ann Cvetkovich, Sara Ahmed and many others have pointed out – from differential biases in each case – there is a *political dimension of affects*, or as I prefer to say: a *political economy of affects* made invisible by this heterosexual, bourgeois, white, Eurocentric-colonial matrix.
>
> On the other hand, as Helena López points out in the Prologue to Sara Ahmed's *La política cultural de las emociones*, it will be a matter of resisting a certain queer voluntarism, a voluntarism that I will call naïve. Not to anchor ourselves in a determinism but to include potency and diminution of potency, possibility and impossibility, in our existences in multiple affectations.

It is within this "queer voluntarism", of which Helena López lucidly warns us, that I locate a non-heterosexual love.

More than one psychoanalyst has replied to me: "but I find in the analysis of gay or lesbian or even trans people, the same difficulties with love as in heterosexual people", to which I invariably reply – a little hartxed by now – "those who subscribe to the *heterosexual device of love* encounter the same difficulties as anyone else. That is why it is a device, because it produces what it was invented for".

Someone who seems to me to know very clearly that this is something else among those who desert the devices of normalisation is Jean Genet. Let us hear him say once again about his erotic-deliquential, abject wanderings: "My talent will be the love I feel for everything that makes up the world of prisons and prisons" (Genet, 2004); curiously enough, I note that this paradoxical love takes devices and not subjects as its object.

Later on, he will say of his writing as an asceticism: "I am putting these notes together for some young people. I would like them to be considered as the consignment of an asceticism among all the delicate ones. The experience is painful and I have not yet finished it". I like to think that this asceticism includes the effects of a normalisation of affective normalisation via love as a device. Genet aspires to what he calls "a moral solitude", and for that it is necessary to break with "the most solid bonds of the world: the bonds of love".

It is through Didier Eribon (2004) in *A Morality of Minority* that I learnt of Patrick Chamoiseau's (1997) term *sentimentality*: that which dominated individuals construct in order to "escape the colonisation of their spirit". This *sentimenteca*, as an alternative invention to the dominant sentimentality, and as an other sentimental education or, better still, as *another erotic imagination/imagery*, goes along the same lines as my need to drop some signifiers of the hetero experience that only forcibly cover what is lived in a non-heterosexual life.

For Genet there is no doubt that there are two *worlds* that do not cover each other, do not coincide, are opposed: that of the *normal* and his own, that of *abjection*. And he writes for both, as Eribon rightly points out:

> The fact that he writes for a small number of imaginary and ideal, "young" and "invested" readers, the real addressees of his books, and thus contributes to constituting them as a "community", in no way prevents Genet from addressing other readers whom he never ceases to rebuke and whom he describes as belonging to the dominant world, which he calls "your world", that is, *the world from which he has been excluded and against which he has had to form himself as a person and as a subject . . . within a literary (and political) strategy which consists of opposing two worlds: the world of the young and the world of the young, the world of the young, the world of the young and the world of the young.)* within the literary (and political) strategy of opposing two worlds: the world to which he belongs (that of abjection) and that of "normal" people (for whom outcasts are "abjects").

I am interested in pointing out or rescuing that of *a world against which he has had to form himself as a person and as a subject*, because it will be Didier Eribon (2017) himself who, in *Society as verdict*, will make visible the way in which injury produces the subject. It does not affect him, it produces him. And this is a line that I intend to continue working on: the violent production of subjects or, to put it more lyrically, the production of *subjects of violence* in its multiple forms and modes.

Not long ago, I asked at a psychoanalysis meeting:

How do you think a subject whose eroticism is an insult to the rest is constituted? Insult in the literal sense: *cocksucker, broken arse, mammadera,* do you think that this is indifferent when it comes to subjective division or to thinking of shame as a lack of being or homosexuality as a defence against paranoia? Or when it comes to claiming identity inconsistency or subjective destitution?

There is also a diversity of positions when it comes to demanding social and political change. I find myself, not by choice or transgressive enjoyment but by subjective survival – believe it or not – among those of us who feel it necessary to maintain an important degree of *illegitimacy*, of non-cooptation, of marginality, of opacity, of the irreplaceable, reconcilable, with respect to a cisheterocapitalist world that does not cease to swallow us up, including us.

Among gay writers, there is considerable variety in the degree of problematisation or naturalisation and inadvertent adoption of the term *love* to describe their erotic practices. From this biased, interested, tendentious, and wounded reading, I like to think that "the love that dare not speak its name", by Oscar Wilde (2016), refers to the fact that love is not its name, and even that having wanted to make a love story out of his relationship with Lord Alfred Douglas was what, in the end, led him to prison. Or that when Pedro Lemebel (2018) writes *No tengo amigos, tengo amores*, by extending love in this unlimited way he makes it disappear or lose consistency, he makes it stagger in its metaphysics.

Notes

1 For the meaning of this term, see the Diccionario de la Real Academia Española: *engrupir*. transitive verb cono sur. To make someone believe by words or actions what is not true. Similar: to deceive.

2 *Degénero, degenerado*, emerged as a curatorial proposal for the exhibition Arte degenerado that we did at the Engelman-Ost Collection in 2015, together with Fabricio Guaragna, C. Lenkiewicz, Caro Sobrino, María Mascaró and Yudi Yudoyoko.

3 This text was originally a paper in the framework of the Cycle *Analysts in the Polis. Gender and abject discourses* (Montevideo, 2015).

4 Daniel Gerber (2012). A (necessary) critique of the notion of gender from psychoanalysis. This reminded me of an anecdote from a moment in Lacan's relationship with Françoise Dolto, in which, as a result of I don't know what kind of interlude or difference, Dolto wrote to Lacan: "Let's please elucidate the ambiguity", to which Lacan replied: "Never!

5 The radical nature of this statement was recently relativised in conversation with Sandra Filippini and Diego Nin, so I would reformulate it – at my own expense, of course – as

"a power that does not exercise but operates in analysis", a formulation that I will not be able to develop here.

6 This text was written on the occasion of the Colloquium "Erotique de la domination. Gamas del acto", at the École Lacanienne de Psychanalyse. Montevideo, 2014.

7 Here we should remember that Jacques Lacan has troubled psychoanalysis in many ways: from his revisiting-revision of the very notion of the unconscious, of analysis as an act, of the symptom, by putting resistance on the side of the analyst, and so on. In the same way – or in other ways – Deleuze and Guattari questioned the familialist drift of psychoanalysis, the Oedipus, and so on. And Foucault – with his notion of the psi function and of the dispositif of sexuality – remains today an annoying fly that does not make life easy for a psychoanalysis that does not want to join in the normalisation of the subjects.

8 Lacan once said that he had never seen two analysts together; there is a logical impossibility there.

9 We have known for some time now – thanks to feminisms – that the personal is political. I propose to reformulate this phrase as: *the singular is political*. This does not imply annulling its singularity, but making it the effect of power devices.

10 Of a power that is not exercised (p. 36).

11 *Degeneradx* is the term I chose to say, appropriating the insult as much as to allude to a possible escape from the sex-generic system: degenerate.

12 In this sense, I find highly recommendable the work of Facundo Saxe (2018): "The death trap: queer drifts from sexual dissidence in the production of scientific knowledge to the infantile memory of a kiss. Etcetera." There Saxe asks, "Can first-person enunciations, our enunciations, or the recovery of our self-histories and our psychic archives, ways of constructing theory and scientific, cultural and philosophical reflection on the basis of those lives that we could not or would not let us see?" And at another point: "Why can't our memories be theory, or our readings, or our lives as theory?"

13 If I hid the copy of the thesis from myself, it is possible that this is due to the shame I feel today about the expert position I assumed at the time, determining who could and who could not have access to the so-called Sex Reassignment Surgery.

14 Facundo Saxe (2018) quote 9, p. 53.

15 In the "Preface to the English edition of Seminar xi", Lacan states: "the unconscious is real, if you believe me", which seems to me to reveal the ambiguity to be sustained.

16 Lacan plays with "hontologie" by combining honte: shame, and ontologie: ontology. Enric Berenguer and Miquel Bassols translate: vergonzontology. Cf. Lacan [1969–70] 1992).

17 *Otherism* would be the current that affirms the past-present discontinuity as opposed to continuism.

18 Halperin analyses and takes as an object of study the queer in the gay as something that defines what he will call his "cultural practices".

19 Perhaps it is necessary to say that Deleuze-Guattari separate schizophrenia as a desiring production from what they call: "the artificial schizophrenic", "as we see it in the hospital, an autistic rag produced as an entity".

20 See *The Anti-Oedipus*, op. cit., p. 24.

21 I play with the idea of dissident or diverse – as well as amusing – versions of the father.

22 See Horacio Etchegoyen (2014).

23 Actually, in the case of Chapulin colorado, the phrase that triggers the appearance of the absurd superhero – no more absurd than any hero, of course – is: "and now who will be able to defend me? Surely, as I am reluctant to be so helpless, I prefer help to defence".

24 I refer to the case of Erns Kris, about a phantom of plagiarism, of which Lacan will give nine versions or readings of it, but particularly to the review by Allouch (2000) – on the occasion of the publication of *El idioma de los lacanianos* by Jorge Baños Orellana – in which he points out the risks of falling into understanding in analysis.

25 Years later, I would become intensely and insistently interested in blackness, the racialisation of bodies, racism, and Afrodiasporic spirituality – which, incidentally, includes non-gendered, degendered entities, and sexual dissident practitioners. Nigerian theorist Oyèronké Oyewùmi (2017) points out in her book *The Invention of Women* that the Yoruba pantheon was not initially sex-gendered. It was colonisation that gave this spirituality its Western and other biases.

26 Only very recently has class oppression begun to be reconsidered in queer theory as a category that cannot be separated from other oppressions, such as gender and race. Likewise in France, Didier Eribon and Édouard Louis, post-foucaultians, brought the issue to the discussion from their autofictional testimonies.

27 I allude ironically to Lacan's idea of Desire of the mother-crocodile and the so-called "maternal ravage", which I believe we should problematise, today more than ever, feminisms notwithstanding.

28 Today I suppose it would be his fur coat, with which he is seen in period photos.

29 The word *magnet* has a multiple etymology full of resonances: aimant-que con- sounds with amant-amante, but it is also something magnetic and a guide, etc.

30 The Lacanians, he said, in the masculine. Even today we still hear "the Lacanians", "the analyst", "the analysand". The woman does not exist. She is made to non-exist.

31 It is in this sense that Gayle Rubin (1975) will say that psychoanalysis is "frustrated feminist theory".

32 I allude to Descartes and his demand for "clear and distinct ideas". I was recently rereading the first volume of *The Hundred Years' Battle. History of psychoanalysis in France.* Vol. 1 (1885–1939), by E. Roudinesco, I find that in the introduction of psychoanalysis in France, one of the pioneers – Angelo Louis Marie Hesnard, a very singular character – bets that the too heterogeneous Freudian theory will be purified by a Cartesian France: "It would be interesting to do an archaeology of this idea of *clarity* from its origins, passing through racism, constituting scientific discourse and permeating a certain psychoanalysis".

33 Theme from the album *En directo*, recorded at the Teatro de verano in Montevideo, 1989 and at Obras sanitarias, Buenos Aires, in 1991. https://es.wikipedia.org/wiki/En_directo_(%C3%A1lbum_de_Patricio_Rey_y_sus_Redonditos_de_Ricota)

34 It is enough to see what Lacan does by trafficking Marx's surplus value into the Freudian field, in the plus-de-jouir. There is there the warning of an economy of jouissance, which is not only not outside the economic system in which we live, but which finds its limit there. See Barrios, F. and Filippini, S. (2021).

35 See Miller, G. "Rendez- vous chez Lacan": https://www.youtube.com/watch?v=9X- vfb8mpp18

36 Available at https://es.wikipedia.org/wiki/Mierda_de_artista

37 It is said of a gift that it brings hidden harm. The Trojan horse is the best known example.

38 The idea belongs to Viveiros de Castro and Deborah Danowski (2019).

39 Incidentally, this colonial, civilising, Eurocentric, and racist mode – let's remember that barbarism is the original peoples in the conquest – persists in authors such as Isabelle Stengers herself, whose subtitle of her book *In Times of Catastrophe* is *How to resist the coming barbarism?*

Chapter 2

Of books

From the wardrobe to psychoanalysis:.[1] On *Gay Oedipus:. Heteronormativity and psychoanalysis* by Jorge N. Reitter

Dedicated to three women – in a micropolitical gesture, since we suppose them to be close, even intimate with the author – and to the homosexual liberation movement, *Gay Oedipus* bursts onto the scene of texts that question psychoanalysis in a double movement: from the inside and from the outside. Or perhaps it would be better to say, from the inside with an outside that problematises, deconstructs – not necessarily in a Derridean way – and puts psychoanalysis in crisis. A psychoanalysis that is traversed, some will say, constituted, others will say, has contributed something no less – discourse – to heteronormativity, I will say.

In an ingeniously and provocatively titled Foreword: "Homophobia in the Closet", it gets straight to the point. Institutional psychoanalysis has kept its homophobia in the wardrobe, but this has not prevented it from denying entry to homosexual analysts.

> On 1 December 1921 Ernst Jones commented in one of the circulars of the Secret Committee that the Dutch had consulted him on the advisability of accepting as a member of the psychoanalytic society 'a doctor manifestly known to be a homosexual'. Jones advised against it, and asked the other members of the Committee whether the exclusion of homo-sexuals from analytic training should be the general rule for the International Psychoanalytic Association. Freud and Rank say no, "the decision in such cases should be based on an individual assessment of the qualities of the person". To my great disappointment, Ferenczi's position (he, who before his encounter with
>
> The first thing that psychoanalysis had bravely defended the rights of "uranists" before the Budapest Medical Association) is that "for the time being it would be better to reject on principle all overt homosexuals; they are generally too abnormal". In the end, the position of denying homosexuals the possibility of psychoanalytic training triumphed, although Freud did not oppose this decision with the firmness with which he defended "profane" analysis. This position prevailed in the I.P.A. for more than fifty years, but it *was never written down*.
>
> (Reitter, 2019)

DOI: 10.4324/9781003710295-2

The expression "too abnormal" would perhaps suffice to give an account of where the interpretive phenomenological analysis (IPA) ideals were going. An unwritten decision suggests the Kafkaesque nature of an ideological imbroglio in which psychoanalysis placed its normative position. Jean Allouch (1996) will call it quality.

Lacan seems to have situated things differently, although this does not guarantee – nothing guarantees almost anything in analysis, it must be said – a shift towards what would eventually be a non-normative psychoanalysis.

Reitter (2019) says:

> I do not have the impression that Lacan's liberality in the factual has been transferred to the Lacanian institutions. I remember, for example, that in my years as a student in the Faculty of Psychology at the UBA (a faculty which in that post-dictatorship climate was experiencing a Lacanian euphoria) the question was raised as to whether a homosexual, a "pervert" according to Lacan, could be a psychoanalyst. That was several years ago, but just a few days ago I was told that Jorge Alemán asked, in a seminar, in which psychoanalytic society members who were gay could be openly gay.

Reitter's style, at times testimonial, always implied, takes up a gesture that I consider no small part of so-called queer literature: one speaks only *from the wound*; *to "speak wounded"*, Daniel Lourenco will say in a Facebook post in 2018. This entails the inconvenience of *speaking for* or *about* others, a lesson that not all have learned, not without costs for those who are thus objectified.

Reitter puts it bluntly:

> Theoretical production in psychoanalysis does not usually emerge from pure and disinterested science (if any science is): it includes the subject and his desire. This book is the journey, the product and the testimony of sustained and intense subjective work (and painful mourning) to resolve questions that no psychoanalysis could solve. Thus, while most of what it says is transferable to other forms of sexual diversity, it is especially focused on the gay question.

Some of this is at play in Fabrice Bourlez's (2018) recommendation in *Queer psychanalyse*. Given that the heterosexuality of the analyst is assumed as evidence, a kind of performative *coming-out* will be necessary before the analysand who claims to be non-heterosexual. To say oneself, to present oneself as a homo-analyst or queer-analyst would be, Bourlez understands, modes of ironic reappropriation of the assumed identities within psychoanalysis (Bourlez, 2018).

To train a queer analyst as one more of the semblants to be brought into play in the analysis if that were necessary? One or two questions insist in *Gay Oedipus:*

> Can one find less heteronormative ways of approaching the relation of the Oedipus complex to the castration complex (as I intend to demonstrate in this book, the heteronormative devices by excellence of psychoanalysis)?

And these questions will be the backbone of the essayistic discourse in chapters that include: “Gay Oedipus”, “Psychoanalysis and homophobia”, “Heteronormativity of psychoanalysis”, “The original entanglement”, “How psychoanalysis could not escape heteronormativity”, “Oedipus reloaded”, “Psychoanalysis and homophobia”, “How psychoanalysis could not escape heteronormativity”, as well as a Miscellany: “On the political incorrectness of eroticism”, “Rethinking the possible as such”, “Homosexuality as disturbance and as luxury”, “Faith Julius Boehm”, and a *bonus track*: “Cycle of conversations ‘to be an analyst’”, a space coordinated by Pablo Tajman and Manuel Murillo, and an “Epilogue”.

A first critical consideration is that of keeping the Oedipus at the centre of the discussions, even once it has been revealed as a normalising device. The objection stems from the Foucauldian warning about devices: a device only enables that for which it was created. I understand, however, that given that the history of *queer* is the history of reappropriations, the attempt is valid.

In the Prologue to the second edition, along with considerations that deal with the coloniality of knowledge and the realisation of its effects on writing – among other things the relative ignorance of other South American voices that are also, we are, trying to say something about it – Reitter lucidly asks himself the following question:

> In the book I insist on visualising a specificity of the *gay experience*, but I also insist on pointing out that what determines that specificity is not subjective, but political. Is there a specificity of the lgttbi clinic? Yes and no. The place that each subject occupies in power relations determines to a large extent his or her subjectivity. In an imaginary non-heteronormative world, a world where *gay Oedipus* would no longer be necessary, the subjectivity of lgttbi people would undoubtedly be different. In such a world, the *gay experience*, for example, would not be determineted by insult and the wardrobe. But surely the forms of sociability and the mode of sex-affective relations of the collective would maintain some specificity, not comparable to the way in which they are established in heterosexuality. Would heterosexuality, as we know it, still exist in that imaginary world? Impossible questions to answer.

To conclude that it is impossible to give an answer seems to me to be a sign of the most analytical aspect of the question. What else is psychoanalysis about if not impossibility? Above all, because to respond would be to fall back into some kind of universal. Nevertheless, we must not let slip the bet on a situated psychoanalysis, which does not ignore the real effects of the historical modes of production of subjects, as well as the effects of injury and discrimination on the basis of which dissident, non-heteronormative subjectivities are constructed.

We call this review “From the psychoanalytic wardrobe. From the closet to psychoanalysis”, convinced that something is at stake there, in this un-placing, which is an act. Reitter poses it as the task of clearing heteronormative ballast, a task that prepares the field for the analytic operation.

There is an operation to be done each time with these ballast so that there is some analysis. And it seems to me an act of justice that one of the epigraphs, alongside those of Foucault and Eve Kosofsky-Sedgwick, is by Monique Wittig, who represents the best of a feminism without which little progress would have been made in questioning heterosexuality as a political regime:

> [T]here remains at the heart of this culture a nucleus of nature that resists examination, a relation excluded from the social in the analysis and which has a character of ineluctability in culture as in nature: it is the heterosexual relation. I would call it the socially obligatory relation between "man" and "woman".

Reitter anticipates criticisms that he knows will follow his book:

> With regard to gayness, my impression is that psychoanalysis tends to take one of two positions (sometimes the same analyst holds both!): either "homosexuality" is a pathology, or it is not a subject. And while I agree that gay, or "homosexual", are not categories of psychoanalysis, I think there is a specificity to the gay experience, which a psychoanalyst would do better to take into account when considering the gay experience.
>
> I think there is a specificity to the gay experience, which a psychoanalyst would do better to take into account when listening to a homosexual person. By "gay experience" I mean the experience that someone goes through just because he or she is gay, regardless of any other subjective considerations.

This resonates for me with some of David Halperin's (2015) insights in *How to be Gay*. regarding both the homosexual experience and the way of *doing* with suffering, another way of doing with:

> [T]he Fire Island widows (gay men who have lost their partners to HIV-Aids and perform Italian widows) laugh first and foremost at their own affliction. When they laugh at horrifying or tragic situations, it is not that they are unaware of the horror or tragedy involved, on the contrary. They laugh because they don't want to laugh, so as not to indulge in maudlin self-pity. But that is not the only thing, for the affliction does not disappear when they laugh at it, if anything it becomes more acute, more concrete. However, it is thus confined to a specific area, a specific social and emotional location, which means that it becomes less constricting, less isolating. As a result, one does not escape from grief, but shares it in a way that enables one to cope with it. Or you "try something" as one of the Amazon commentators reminds us of Faye Dunaway as Joan Crawford. Esther Newton sums it up: "humour doesn't cover up, it transforms". Hence the statement that: "camp drains the suffering of a pain it does not seek to conceal". This explains why horror can coexist with humour in the poetics of gay discourse . . . parody without the slightest implication of cruelty, distancing or denial.

There is, for Halperin, a poetics of gay discourse that drains the suffering of pain.

I recently tried to locate how Jean Genet, in all his work, had shown other ways of doing with what one lives, with what one suffers, not only in the field of art but in life itself. Thus, for example, betrayal could be the greatest act of love in the face of the loss of the beloved. A kind of erotic-amorous asceticism that opens another way to mourning as an act.

And although Lacan says that anguish does not lie, there is a performativity in the production of affects, a heteroperformativity, a dramaturgy that often hinders the possibility of making room for the singular, very singular drifts that each person makes with what affects them. And this radical nature of the singular makes all pathologising pretensions fall, as long as they are accepted.

This does not mean annulling the complex relation singularity-political dimension in the production of subjects. I could paraphrase feminism by saying: *The singular is political*, and in this discursive operation neither term cancels the other but implies it. So there will be, for example, a lot of material to cut through in this revisiting of so-called homosexuality, starting from the duo that has been evident for some psychoanalysis up to now: paranoia-homosexuality. The psychologisation of power relations and their dispositives only gives them consistency, reality.

Reitter says:

> A gay man *is* not haunted by his gayness, in many areas he is; he is not, or is not just a neurotic phantasm. If we think of it only in terms of "psychological" mechanisms, we only reinforce the power arrangements that impose silence on the subject.

Reitter is critical of certain psychoanalytical refrains that are repeated and emptied of any critical view. The *case-by-case* approach, for example, can suffer from this drift:

> If everything could be reduced to questions of the subject, his or her desire, to a subject that is thus reduced to the individual, if a "case-by-case" approach were sufficient, as if everyone could do what he or she wanted in absolute (not determined) terms, why was it that for such a long period of time no one spoke out and then the voices multiplied rapidly? It is clear that a change in historical circumstances (i.e., power relations) made it possible to speak out.

And since it would be impossible to say everything that is said in this book, I will end by alluding to what seems to me to be a central point in any contemporary debate that proposes a necessary detachment from heteronormativity: sexual difference, this "nucleus of nature", to paraphrase Wittig, which claims to be a pre-discursive reality. Difference, which authors as diverse as Paul B. Preciado (2019b) and Oyeronké Oyewumi (2017) agree in considering constitutive of the West. A politico-visual system, Preciado will say. Logic, bio-logic, visual, Oyewumí will say. Oedipus, castration, phallus are its main psychoanalytical derivations.

Reitter says:

> In general, theorists in gay and lesbian studies violently reject the whole supposedly phallocentric approach of psychoanalysis, and I think with good reason: how could they not reject an approach that says that they are sick, that they have not reached mature, genital sexuality, that leaves them on the side of perversion or of the "unhappy" solutions of the Oedipus complex? In my opinion, they are quite right in their rejection, and at the same time there is much truth in the Freudian approach to the phallus as the computer of sexual jouissance. The question is how to free the theorisation of the phallic phase from the ballast that renders it heteronormative.

It seems to me that the issue is precisely there, in not realising that the so-called phallus can be – in fact, it is – *an* author of sexual jouissance, which patriarchal societies, historically regulated by sexual difference, the sex-gender system, and heterosexuality as a political regime, have given themselves as the only one. Reitter points to the possibility of a *degeneration* of the Edipo, which also implies the *acceptance* of sexual difference even if not its *choice* of sexual partner. Although interesting, I am less optimistic about this because I understand that sexual difference-sex-gender system and compulsory heterosexuality exclude any other possible drift.

In this sense, I find Jean Allouch's work on the *non-sexual relation* equally promising, which could finally at least make the idea of castration unnecessary. This does not necessarily drop sexual difference, which remains present, even if it has become a position, a side, in the formulas of sexuation. Unless it is risked that there is no sexual relation, as long as there is no writing of the sexual, it derives from the fact that *there is no sexual* outside its signifying existence. This is why I believe that we still have to continue working for psychoanalysis to become an erotology of passage. Eros and logos will still have to be revised in the quest for another regulation, for the diverse, and not for difference and binarism. In that sense, I find it more than encouraging that books such as *Gay Oedipus* continue to summon us to escape from all normativity.

The power of a tremor: Notes on *An apartment on Uranus: Chronicles of the crossroads* by Paul B. Preciado

> My trans condition is a new form of uranism. I am not a man. I am not a woman. I am not hetero-sexual. I am not homosexual. I am not bi-sexual either. I am a dissident of the sex-gender system. I am the multiplicity of the cosmos locked in a binary epistemological and political regime, screaming in front of you. I am a Uranist in the confines of techno-scientific capitalism.
>
> —Paul B. Preciado

Inadvertence

Some may wonder about the status of this writing, about its genre, and it would not be entirely wrong. For some time now my writing, along with my life – or in reverse order, it matters little – has been degenerating. Having been born and raised in the literate culture and literature that still maintained its generic boundaries, barely expanded or distended, and after many years of academic teaching and pretendedly scientific writing, something of that way of saying – or of writing, as saying by other means – was no longer sustained.

The first realisation of this was the rejection of an article by the Revista de la Sociedad de Psiquiatría del Uruguay with the argument: "writing with features of an unacceptable orality for an academic communication". That was my last attempt to continue to fit in with writing formats that had not welcomed me for a long time. Then it was no longer possible to maintain the dissociation: poetic writing-academic or psychoanalytical or essayistic or journalistic writing, and, at the risk of an indigestible and indigestible *melange*, it was necessary to invent other ways of saying-writing that hack into editorial and/or disciplinary devices.

All this is to say that these are notes, somewhere between review and commentary, between article and semblance, between essay and discursive appropriation, between neologisation of what has already been neologised and quotation. Between textual performance and plagiarism.

In-advertidx (warned that reading is writing) that what is read is written, is said, making the text say what it (does not) say, in a sort of cannibalistic appropriation that prevents us from sparing ourselves the singularity of all reading. Here we go . . .

Chronicles of the Crossroads

> If this book is written under the sign of Uranus, it is because it contains some of the "chronicles of the crossroads". These are the chronicles, texts mostly written in airports and hotel rooms, which I wrote for the French newspaper *Libération* and for some other European media between 2010 and early 2018. . . . This is also the sequence of this sexual and gender transition, the story of the crossing.
>
> (Preciado, 2019b)

This is how Paul B. Preciado, at another point on a path whose beginning could be placed pharmaco-writorially in *Testo yonki* (Preciado, 2008); testotexto conceived as: "an autofiction . . . a protocol of voluntary intoxication based on synthetic testosterone that concerns the body and the affections of B. P. . . . a bodily essay". Text written between two important shocks for B. P.: the death of Guillaume Dustan and his falling in love – "tropismo", as he calls it – with Virginie Despentes.

As I have written many times before, it is no longer possible to avoid discursive implication. It will be necessary to show one's true colours and to accept the testimonial slant that underlies all writing. The chronicles begin as a manifesto – in the knowledge that this modernist gesture is destined to obsolescence, but without for that reason dropping its decisive power, its political *poiesis*. Manifesto dediced, not, as might be expected, to the rising right but to "the left-wing gurus of old colonial Europe",

> who stubbornly want to explain to the activists of the Occupy movement, the 15-M movement, the transfeminists of the crippled-trans-whore-maric-bollero-intersex and post-porn movement that we cannot make the revolution because we don't have an ideology. They say "an ideology" as my father used to say *a husband.*
>
> (Preciado, 2008)

This allusion to the supposed absence of ideology in the framework of the opposite adjudication by those who situate queer-transfeminism as "gender ideology" (Márquez and Lage, 2016) is interesting. The (European) left and right seem to be in unison, perhaps for different reasons, but with the common reason of not being able to docilely add dissidents, gender defectors, to their party ranks.

From B. P. to P. B., much more has happened than a simple substitution or alteration in the order of the letters. And I could also say that nothing substantial has happened, insofar as we are not dealing with substances – well, we are dealing with substances, but not ontological ones – but with somatopolitical fictions and cyborg pharmaco-identities.

What is interesting is that they are chronicles of the crossroads, insofar as they are traversed by Paul B. Preciado's transition. Preciado's transition, which is not the same as saying that they speak *of* it but *from* there, or in that intersection, a meeting of forces and multiple flows. Between them. Between, for example: "the relations between private and public spaces, between property and the commons, between truth and secrecy, between politics and pornography", as he will say in the chronicle dedicated to the Julian Assange affair (Preciado, 2008).

It is enough to look at the Table of Contents to see the miscellany of places from which Paul B. chooses or is led to fabricate these chronicles that are also chronicles of his time and the events of this global political transition: "Decimos revolución", "El último cercamiento: Aprendiendo de la deuda con Silvia Federici", "Goteras diplomáticas: Julian Assange and the Sexual Limits of the Nation-State", "Derrida, Foucault and Impossible Biographies", "Filiation and Queer Love according to Jean Genet", "Veiled Revolutions: Simone de Beauvoir's Turban and Arab Feminism", "Who Defends the Queer Child?" "Politically assisted procreation and state hetero-sexualism", "Candy Crush or addiction in the age of telecommunication", etc.

Or it could be said in another way, which is never without consequences: it is about a transition and crossings that are not individual, that do not happen to isolated subjects but that happen in a planned way, that take place globally, mutating bodies and devices and migrant identities, escaping in a diverse and convergent way at least at some points of crossing.

> Sex change and migration are the two crossing practices that, by questioning the political and legal architecture of patriarchal colonialism, sexual difference and the nation-state, place a living human body at the limits of citizenship and even of what we understand as humanity.
>
> (Preciado)

Paul B. is not alone in this micropolitical uprising:

> In every corner of the world, from Athens to Kassel, from Rojava to Chiapas, from São Paulo to Johannesburg, it is possible to feel not only the exhaustion of traditional forms of doing politics, but also the emergence of hundreds of thousands of practices of social, sexual, political, artistic experimentation. . . . In the face of the uprising of oedipal and fascist powers, micro-politics of crossing over are emerging everywhere.

Nevertheless, against the tide of those who claim that queer is an absence of suffering, an absence of symptom, the lack that cannot be missing, the transition and the crossing over will not be without commotion, without risk. And although the old psychopathological jargon demands to speak of anguish or symptom, this will be said in other ways; other jargons, other grammars will have to be tried out if we want to stop saying the same thing. For as David Halperin (2015) shows us in *How to be Gay*, there are alternatives to the "heterosexual dramaturgy of affects".

Nor, by the way, will it be a matter of mere pharmacopornographic consumption, but rather one that, when used politically, makes its biopolitical character visible.

> The decision to "change sex" is necessarily accompanied by what Édouard Glissant calls "a tremor". The crossroads is the place of uncertainty, of non-evidence, of the strange. And as this is not a debility, but a potency. . . . To "change sex" is not, as the guard of the old sexual regime would have it, a leap into psychosis. But neither is it, as the new neoliberal management of sexual difference pretends, a mere medical-legal procedure that can be completed during puberty to give way to an absolute normality.

Of Western religiosity and science fiction, Paul B. will take up, without saying so, the warning about Western and capitalist religiosity already pointed out by Max Weber ([1905] 2004) and Walter Benjamin (1985), among others, and will highlight, via science, one of its hard cores or blind spots, depending on how you want to see it: sexual difference. "If the heteropatriarchal regime of sexual difference is the scientific religion of the West, then changing sex can only be a heretical act" (Preciado, 2008).

It will then be a heresy-act articulated in more than one movement; "shamanic rituals" in a literal and metaphorical sense, somewhat reminiscent of Alejandro Jodorowsky's psychomagical acts. If capitalism is black magic, as Tiqqun (1999) and The Invisible Committee taught us, *anti-capitalist magic* that subverts the spell(s) will be indispensable.[2]

The change of name will become inevitable in this passage from one identity fiction to another, as one more hacking of the system. Change of voice – in the material-phonological sense and in the sense of a decisive and scriptural voice – and change of name will not be without setbacks, which will include false steps such as trying to take the name of Subcomandante Marcos, the Zapatista leader, and becoming only fleetingly so: Beatriz Marcos. Until January 2016, when Paul B. will take over the fictional signature.

> That when I started a series of magical rituals to find a name, I set out to do what I needed to do to change. I gave myself over to the crossroads. That's how, at last, I dreamt my new name one night in December 2015 in a bed in the Gothic Quarter of Barcelona[3]: I accepted the name, strangely and absurdly. I took it as my own. I asked the whole world to call me by that name. At the same time, I started a legal process to demand a change of name and legal sex.
>
> (Preciado, 2008)

Magic, dreams, shamanic rituals, pharmacopolitical initiations and multiple becomings, together with philosophical-political analysis and anti-colonial, artistic-curatorial activism, not without rock-star positions, will be enabled as tools in an expanded and always open box. Tools of de-knowledge, asceticism of the self.

> I wanted to become unknown. . . . I didn't ask for testosterone from medical institutions as a hormonal therapy to cure a supposed "gender dysphoria". I wanted to function with testosterone, to produce the intentionality of my desire in connection with it, to multiply my faces by metamorphosing my subjectivity, to make a body as one makes a revolutionary machine.
>
> (Preciado, 2008)

To function with, to make a machine, to become an agency, the politics of the cyborg, the promise of monsters. And as in *La invención del género, o el tecnocordero que devora a los lobos (*Preciado, year), "el saber del tecnocordero engaña a la manada de lobos", some of the medical and legal knowledge-power is mocked, hacked, by another "lesser" knowledge, with the tools of the master – used in another way, re-appropriated, expropriated.

Something of a plunge into a trans-mutant material unconsciousness – unconsciousness noticed, lucid dreaming – will give rise to de-identifications[4] and dis-identifications of the self, to de-fictionalisations[5] and only temporary, positional, relational re-fictionalisations as a politics of the multiple.

> Over the years, I have learned to consider dreams, whether for comfort or wisdom, as an integral part of life. There are dreams which, because of their sensory intensity, sometimes because of their realism and sometimes, precisely, because of their lack of realism, deserve to belong to a biography with the same right as the most notorious of the events that took place during what we commonly reduce to what we understand as truly lived experiences, i.e., those that occur during wakefulness. After all, life begins and ends in unconsciousness, so that the actions that we carry out in full consciousness are but islets in an archipelago of dreams.
>
> (Preciado, 2008)

Something of a speculative empowerment, of a disbelief in scientific religiosity, emerges in and from different voices. Donna Haraway (2018) and her notion of speculative fabulation is, perhaps, one of the most heard today, at the risk of not recognising in her a genealogy that includes Isabelle Stengers,[6] Ursula Le Guin, and so many others who dare to dissociate themselves from this, a prized commodity in Western hegemonic rationality.

In fact, a psychoanalysis that claims to be Lacanian would have trouble being swallowed up by scientific discourse. In this field, too, the relation to science and the scientific cannot remain unproblematised. *Not without* science and its Cartesian subject, the Cartesian cogito is not subverted, not being there where it is thought.[7]

> (2) a reflection on the relation between forms of oppression and forms of formal understanding or theory building; (3) an emerging redefinition of marginality as a location, of its identity as a disidentification and (4) the hypothesis of self-displacement which expresses the simultaneous social, subjective, internal and external movement, which is in reality a political and personal movement". In this regard, see: "Eccentric Subjects: Feminist Theory and Historical Consciousness" by Teresa de Lauretis in María C. Cangiamo and Lindsay DuBois (eds., 1993) and José Esteban Muñoz (1999).

However, Paul B. does not bet on psychoanalysis – as almost none of those who write from the field of sexogenic dissidence do[8] – and perhaps that could be a warning for those of us who still play our cards there: "A technochaman from Pocha Nostra[9] is worth more than a neo-Lacanian psychonegotiant, and a Post-Op contrasexual fisting is better than a protocol vaginoplasty" (Preciado, 2008). Psychoanalysts and protocol surgeons, we still – I want to believe that we can rescue ourselves – suffer the same fate. The same fate that Foucault made us suffer when he placed us on the side of the psi function.

De-eroticising the sexual, desexualising the erotic

In the end, this is an erotic as well as a political gamble:

> Heterosexuality is not only, as Monique Wittig teaches us, a regime of government: it is also a politics of desire. . . . This practice of government does not take the form of a law, but of an unwritten norm, of a transaction of gestures and codes that have the effect of establishing in the practice of sexuality a partition between what can and cannot be done. This form of sexual servitude is based on an aesthetic of seduction, a stylisation of desire and a choreography of pleasure. This regime is not natural: it is a historically constructed and codified aesthetics of domination that eroticises the difference of power and perpetuates it. It is this politics of desire that keeps the old sex-gender regime alive despite the legal processes of democratisation and women's empowerment. This heterosexual

> necropolitical regime is today as degrading and destructive as vassalage and slavery were at the height of the Enlightenment.
>
> (Preciado)

De-eroticising oppression, desiring freedom could be ways towards another eroticism, another politics of desire. Of course, this is where Paul B. Preciado concludes, perhaps something is beginning for us, questions open up: Will we continue to maintain desire as a politics? Will we not make room for Foucault's and Lee Edelman's objections about desire?[10]

On the other hand, with respect to violence, it is not a *naïve* appeal in Preciado:

> I am not saying that queer and transfeminist culture escapes all forms of violence. There is no sexuality without shadow. But it is not necessary for the shadow (inequality and violence) to preside over and determine sexuality.

Despite this, Paul B. maintains here the notion of sexuality, which is a contradiction in terms, insofar as nothing else but the device of sexuality establishes sexual difference. The sexual as a *sex-generic device* – allow me the *match*[11] Foucault-Gayle Rubin – is not without violence.

There are those of us who cannot fail to welcome the power of this fear, of which this writing is but one of its effects.

Notes

1 Jorge N. Reitter. *Oedipo gay. Heteronormativity and psychoanalysis*. Buenos Aires, Letra Viva Editorial, 2019.

2 In the sense of multiple and diverse practices ranging from Postporno to Shibari sessions: erotic bondage or S/M – which erotically subvert power relations – to artistic-political activism or psychomagical acts reappropriated by dissidences. Something of the production of another imaginary, of a radical imagination not without real effects.

3 The account that Paul B. Preciado's account at the presentation of his book at the Les Cahiers de Colette bookshop in Paris in June 2019 of how he came to acquire his new name, Paul, is not to be missed. After having tried to appropriate the name Marcos, a name that the Zapatista subcomandante dropped – his new name: Galeno – when announcing his new name on social networks, he will be criticised as this gesture is interpreted by Latin American activists as a colonial act, Preciado asks his friends to name him – which will not be successful either – until, finally, someone he calls a "tecnochamana" reverses the bet by telling him: "it's not about looking for a name, a name is looking for you". And that name he will find in a dream, long after it was announced to him in a long shamanic ceremony: "I dreamt that I found the complete and secret poetry of Marx . . . and that this forced a total revision of Marx's work . . . and on leaving La Pléiade-Gallimard, a former professor of mine in the US said to me: "Hi, Paul! Do you want to edit the version of Marx's complete works with the poetry with us? in La Pléiade?" This name will later be confirmed by the shaman consulted. This obviously opens up a whole possible chapter in relation to the proper name in the field of psychoanalysis, a chapter which, however, we can only mention here.

4 Here I paradoxically allude to the well-known phrase of the feminist Audre Lorde (1979, cited in Lorde, 2003): "The master's tools will never dismantle the master's house" in *The Sister, the Foreigner. Articles and lectures*.

5 Teresa de Lauretis (1993) and José Esteban Muñoz (1999), from different slants, introduced the subject of disidentifications in the queer field. De Lauretis locates there what he calls the "third moment of feminist theory" and characterises it as "its current stage of reconceptualisation and elaboration of new terms: (1) a reconceptualisation of the subject as a changing entity, which multiplies along diverse axes of difference; (2). A kind of immersion in a transmuting material unconscious – perceived unconscious, lucid dream – will give rise to disidentifications of the self, to defictionalizations and refictionalizations that are only temporary, positional, and relational, as a politics of the multiple.

6 Some of this can be found in Mathieu Rivat and Aurélien Berland (2016).

7 I play here with Jacques Lacan's "I think where I am not . . .".

8 Almost with the sole exception of Lee Edelman (2014) in *No to the Future. La teoría queer y la pulsión de muerte*, although his use of psychoanalysis there is highly singular and to be problematised.

9 La Pocha Nostra is a shifting, transdisciplinary arts organisation, founded in 1993 by Guillermo Gómez Peña, Roberto Sifuentes, and Nola Mariano, in California.

10 In Foucault's case, the objection is linked to the relation desire-lack-repression. Cf. Michel Foucault (1977b), *History of Sexuality. Vol. I, The Will to Know*. In Edelman's case, to what he understands as the reproductive character of all desire, insofar as it is born and sustained by a constitutive lack that is sought to be remedied in an improbable future, which leads him to propose queerness as the impossible project of making oneself unx with jouissance and the death drive, "dismantling the subject from within". Cf. L. Edelman, op. cit. 59.

11 In applications such as Tinder or Grindr, the match is the coincidence of "likes" between two users, which enables contact and chatting. Here the match would be between the sex-gender system of Gayle Rubin, see her article: "The Traffic in Women: A Note on the Political Economy of Sex" (1975), and the question of the dispositif of sexuality in M. Foucault. Sexuality as a sex-gender device – let me quote Foucault and Gayle Rubin together – is not exempt from violence.

Chapter 3

Other spiritualities

Then I said you said we said It is now we said
It is now
And the eye opened like the echo Never heard by Narcissus Like the queen of the night Before the gaze of no one
Of all
Of all that is once Only once and forever Repetitive dream of reptiles
Wise and profoundly ignorant
And the eye was opened For us who fled lightly
And scented for nothing For no one
And in the eye of fear

—Fernando Barrios (unpublished)

Fetishism: Other possible versions that would not be of the father[1]

In the framework of the analysis of the effects of coloniality in psychoanalysis, the spiritual dimension of conquest becomes more and more evident to me. Spiritual coloniality, colonisation of the spirit, colonial spirit.

We are used to consider the passage of languages as a possibility/impossibility of translation or, at best, from an intercultural perspective, integrating the diversity of languages, the colonial gesture becomes an act. Taking a term from another language to designate something of one's own is not without a policy of appropriation. And this is doubled when the chosen term will – after the appropriating gesture – designate negative connotations for the culture of arrival.

Epistemic racism or raciality of the episteme.

If we add to this the fact that in this case fetishism will come to signify a sexual "deviation" or "aberration" with respect to the hetero-norm, the crossing and overlapping of oppressions that intersectionality warns about in the dissident field expands to include a less visible colonial dimension. Fetishism – from the Portuguese *feitico:* "spell", from the Latin *facticius:* "fact", "that which is not natural" – will be one of those terms objectified by colonisation, whose effects of coloniality cut across different cultures. The term is used in a number of fields: sexuality,

DOI: 10.4324/9781003710295-3

psychoanalysis, Marxism, as well as operating in language from a naturalised epistemic raci(on)ality.

José Assandri (2008) points out in his text "La saga del fetichismo":

> The passage of fetishism from century to century, over five centuries, began when certain Portuguese explorers named *feitisso*, "enchanted thing", "bewitched thing", those material objects worshipped by the inhabitants of southern Africa. The conquering enterprise of those Christians led them to stumble upon pieces of roots, shiny stones, bones, which were worshipped by the aborigines if hunting and gathering went well, but destroyed if things went badly. And they found these gods and this treatment strange. But they themselves had long worshipped relics: ashes, bones, locks of hair, teeth and pieces of saints' garments were trafficked all over the Christian world. And they were able to spend fortunes for a piece of cloth that would have been part of the holy shroud, or a piece of wood that was said to have been part of the cross on which the Son of God was nailed. It is said that in the Middle Ages several ships could have been built with the amount of wood that circulated bearing the mark of the cross of Jesus Christ. The Christian explorer, with his relic of the cross in his hand, was unaware of the African who worshipped a piece of root, but couldn't both believers have recognised each other as being of the same wood? The basic argument of fetishism, since then and onwards, has been to mark something as degradation through ignorance.

It was Charles de Brosses, a French magistrate and scholar and contributor to *Diderot and D'Alembert's Encyclopédie or Dictionnaire raisonné des sciences, arts and crafts*, who introduced the term into the West in the eighteenth century. His book *On the Cult of the Fetish Gods*, published in 1760, initiated this colonial genealogy of fetishism. De Brosses set out to analyse a particular kind of religion, which he called *paganas*, the worship of which was directed towards "earthly and material objects called fetishes by the African Negroes . . . and which I shall call fetishism".

He makes it clear that he will also make use of this notion with regard to any other people or nation in which the objects of worship are animals or inanimate beings that are deified, which he considers a belief that is as ancient as it is absurd. He will call them "stupid spirits affected by this passion", "savage peoples who spend their lives in perpetual infancy", "puerile worship", and so on.

A common misunderstanding is to believe that this term comes from those who participate in this rituality, when in fact it is a signifier assigned by the Portuguese colonisers. The colonising gesture is already present in the non-mining itself.

In the nineteenth century, Karl Marx (2001 [1867]) will recolonise the term by producing his famous "commodity fetishism", thus unveiling the magical dimension of capitalism[2] and inadvertently making viable the political operation that had attempted to sustain a Western rationality at the antipodes of primitive and irrational cultures. In Marx, the fetishistic character of the commodity will entail a secret. Hence the title: "The fetishistic character of the commodity and its secret".

> At first glance, a commodity seems an obvious, trivial thing. But its analysis shows it to be a very complex thing, full of metaphysical subtleties and theological quibbles. As a use-value, there is nothing misterious about it. . . . But as soon as it presents itself as a commodity, it is transformed into a sensible, super-sensible thing.

The mystical character of the commodity does not derive from its use-value but from its exchange-value, behind which human labour is hidden. The money form, instead of revealing the social character of labour and social relations, conceals them. Thus, Marx says in an allegory naive: "if commodities could speak they would say . . . we only confront each other as exchange values". The reasons for this fetishistic transformation are to be sought in "the nebulous region of the religious world, in which the products of the human brain seem to be independent beings, endowed with particular bodies and related to each other with men" (Marx, 2001 [1867]).

In the twentieth century, Freud introduced the term *fetishism* into the field of psychoanalysis in the "Essay on sexual aberrations", part of *Three Essays on Sexual Theory*, published in 1905:

> inappropriate substitute for the sexual object. An entirely special aspect is offered by those cases in which the normal sexual object is replaced by another object which is related to it, but is completely inappropriate to serve the normal sexual goal. With a view to classification, it would have been better if we had mentioned this extremely interesting group of aberrations of the sexual drive already when speaking of deviations from the sexual object. But we postponed this until we became aware of the factor of sexual overestimation, on which these phenomena, which lead to an abandonment of the sexual goal, depend.
>
> (Freud, 1993)

The abnormality of this modality is repeatedly pointed out, although a certain degree of fetishism is recognised in erotic-amorous normality, particularly in the stages of infatuation when the normal sexual goal is unattainable or its fulfilment seems to be delayed:

> "Procure me a handkerchief from her bosom, a garter for the love I feel". The pathological case occurs only when the aspiration to the fetish becomes fixed, exceeding the above-mentioned condition, and replaces the normal sexual goal; and furthermore, when the fetish becomes detached from that particular person and becomes a sexual object in its own right. These are the general conditions for mere variations of the sexual drive become pathological deviations. In the choice of the fetish, the persistent

> influence of a sexual impression received almost always in early childhood is manifested – and later abundantly documented – by Binet [1888], who was the first to state this.

In 1927 in "Fetishism" (1986a), Freud will say: "To put it more clearly: the fetish is the substitute for the phallus of the woman (of the mother) in which the little boy has believed and which he does not want to renounce . . . – we know why". It is in this text that Freud adds to dismemberment the splitting of the ego as a key operation for understanding fetishism, but not only that. At the beginning he will call it bi-scission: "If I return to the description of fetishism, I must point out that there are certainly numerous and important proofs of the bi-scission of the fetishist's attitude towards the problem of the castration of the woman".

In an interpretative excess, undoubtedly colonial and universalising, he will say from what he calls the "psychology of peoples":

> Another variant, but at the same time a parallel to fetishism in the psychology of peoples, is the Chinese custom of first mutilating the female foot and then worshipping the mutilated part as a fetish. It is believed that the Chinese man wants to thank the woman for having undergone castration.

Auguste Comte would extend the term to include the worship of the stars and certain people. From his evolutionary perspective of human subjectivity, there would be three stages: a theological or fictitious one, a metaphysical or abstract one, and finally a positive or scientific one, including in the first three phases: fetishism, polytheism, and monotheism.

Lacan, for his part, will keep fetishism in the field of perversion, but not without imprinting on this term another effect of sense – by relying on language – per-version as a version of the father. Subsequently, in an article originally published in English: Fetishism: The Symbolic, the Imaginary and the Real (2015), Lacan, together with Vladimir Granoff, put forward the idea of perversion as a version of the father:

> As Freud recommended, the study of fetishism is and remains most instructive for anyone who focuses on oedipal dynamics in order to understand more fully what the ego is by the egoic split [or] fetishism is born historically, on the demarcation line between anguish and guilt, between the dual and the three-sided relation. Freud does not fail to note this when he recommends the study of fetishism to anyone who might doubt the fear of castration; in the notes following the *Three Essays, he* says that the per- versions are the residue of the development towards the Oedipus complex. For it is here that the various elements that make up instinct can be dissociated.
>
> (Lacan and Granoff, 2015)

Phobia and fetishism will be privileged avenues in the analysis of the object relation, fetishism being the perversion of the perversions, where the anguish in the absence of the phallus in the mother is best shown. The fetish as a symbol of the phallus with which it seeks to disprove castration.

In the Seminar on *Object Relations* ([1956–57] 2007), Lacan will speak of Maya's veil as a curtain:

> The veil, the curtain in front of something, also provides the best illustration of the fundamental situation of love. It can even be said that when the curtain is present, what lies beyond it as a lack tends to be realised as an image. This and no other is the function of a curtain, whatever it may be. The curtain acquires its value, its being and its consistency precisely because absence is projected and imagined on it. The curtain is, shall we say, the idol of absence. If Maya's veil is the most commonly used metaphor to express man's relationship with everything that captivates him, there is no lack of reasons, no doubt, but it is most certainly due to the feeling that there is a certain fundamental illusion in all the relations concocted with his desire. This is where man incarnates, makes an idol, out of his feeling of that nothingness that lies beyond the object of love.

And then there will be possible transitions or drifts:

> It is something behind which the subject is centred. He places himself, not in front of the veil, but behind it, that is to say in the place of the mother, adhering to a position of identification in which the mother needs to be protected, in this case by means of a sheath. This gives us the transition between cases of fetishism and cases of transvestism. The sheath is not like the veil, but a form of protection. It is an aegis with which the subject is wrapped, identified with the female character. Another typical relationship, sometimes particularly exemplary, are the explosions of exhibitionism, in some cases truly reactive, sometimes alternating with fetishism. This is always observed when the subject makes an effort to get out of his labyrinth by reason of a certain staging of the real which leaves him in a position of unstable equilibrium, and there is a crystallisation or inversion of his position.

Fetishism, homosexuality, transvestism, and exhibitionism will become a series. Fetishism and the use of the phallus, one could say in this logic. Just to take two moments in the Lacanian elaboration of the fetish and fetishism, we will say that in the Seminar *Anguish* ([1962–63] 2006b), the fetish has become the object that causes desire:

> The fetish causes desire. Desire, for its part, goes wherever it can. It is not at all necessary for her to be the one wearing the slipper, the slipper can be in her surroundings. It is not even necessary for her to be the bearer of the breast, the breast can be on her head. . . . The fetish is the condition in which her desire is sustained.

Enrique Dussel (1993), for his part, in *Las metáforas teológicas de Marx (Marx's Theological Metaphors)*, among other texts, deals with fetishism. Given that he is someone who was particularly and early on aware of the Eurocentric colonial traversal, one would expect to find in his writing another consideration of the issue. Dussel warns: "The theme of fetishism and religion – like very few other themes – runs through Marx's *entire life*, that is to say, *through his entire work;* which, from the outset, shows us its importance".

From the young Marx, in what he sees as the passage from "Jew and believing layman to critical university student", he quotes:

> The ancient peoples, the savages, among whom the teaching of Christ has not yet been heard, reveal in the *sacrifice (Opfer) of victims to their gods*, in the conviction that through the *sacrifice (Opfer)* they will obtain forgiveness for their sins, an inner uneasiness, fear of the divine wrath and inner conviction of his reprobation.

And these will be false gods, created by the hands of the fetishists. Marx will thus pass, according to Dussel, "from the *political* critique of the Lutheran Christian state to the *economic* critique of fetishism" (Dussel, 1993, p. 41). Finally: "Fetishism will be [for Marx] the alienated essence of man as the negation of community", says Dussel. Likewise, the notion of sacrifice will run through the whole work: the worker will be sacrificed through his labour, the fruit of which no longer belongs to him; alienation, labour for another.

A point that particularly interests Dussel is what he reads as the unnecessary nature of atheism as a requirement for de-alienation. He quotes Marx:

> Atheism, in so far as it denies this lack of essentiality, *is now totally meaningless*, for atheism is the denial of God and affirms, by this denial, the existence of man; but socialism, in so far as it is socialism, no longer needs such mediation. . . . It is *positive* self-consciousness unmediated by the supersession of religion.

And he concludes: "That is to say, from this moment onwards atheism is no longer necessary; socialism is the practical overcoming of such atheism". He compares Marx to Christ and concludes that Marx's critique of religion is "an accurate – and entirely relevant critique from a Christianity of liberation – against the "religion of resignation", of domination, of fetishism.

Here the fetishist term is returned to those who produced it in order to deny validity to others, but it does not function as appropriation since it is reapplied without its necessary problematisation. Subaltern appropriation only operates when it is the offended party who performs it in a gesture of re-signification and value transmutation. That is to say that, here again, I cannot find a warning regarding the adoption of a term that – even though it is not part of the spiritualities that it attempts to name – speaks of other modes of relation between beings and entities, in multiple and diverse agencements of power. Fetishism, animism, paganism and others are signifiers of active, annulling, racist ignorance that invalidates other ways of being in relation, of producing worlds, of making the common.

The obvious question that seems to emerge from this minimal survey of the various vicissitudes of this notion, which is repeatedly a colonial epistemic object, is: what happened or where did the spirituality of other peoples come to play in this other relationship to objects and beings? And even more: how does a ritual practice become a sexual perversion or a feature of capitalist economic production? How does something highly esteemed by some spirits become such a disregard? How does something eminently bearing a spiritual truth become false, deceitful, or demonic? And perhaps not only how does it come about – in various appropriationist and colonial operations – but what consequences does it have on the viability of non-Western, non-Catholic, non-Christian lives, sustained by other spiritual matrices?

There is a word that is missing in this journey, and it is precisely that of those who have been spoken, said by these others, who from the epistemic arrogance that characterises the West, do not cease to make versions of some father, pére-versions.

Why Olodumare is not God. *Work in progress.* Step one: The return of the oppressed

> *ol*: Owner/*odu*: Chapter, power, secret/*mare*: Eternal, constant, constant, fixed, unattainable
>
> Olodumare created the earth along with all living beings, furthermore, he also created all the orishas as his first and greatest children, and appointed the orisha Obatala with the creation of the bodies of mankind; Olodumare then breathed souls into those bodies and from there humanity was born, in time, humans populated the earth and spent all day bothering Olodumare, asking for favours and complaining about their lives, they were noisy, annoying and made the earth a mess. Olodumare grew tired of humanity so he decided to bequeath a part of his ashé to each of his eldest sons, the orishas and gave them dominion over nature, charged the orishas to attend to the affairs of humanity and retired from Earth to continue creating the rest of the universe.[3]

America was never completely Catholic, in spite of the hegemonic pretension of this religion, which was also claimed to be seen as a "Catholic" religion.

Says Mignolo (2007):

> In Europe, Asia and Africa no one knew of the existence of the territory that was to be called the West Indies and later America, nor of the peoples who inhabited it, who would later be known as Indians. America fell from the sky – literally speaking – that Amerigo Vespucci was observing when he discovered that the stars he saw from today's southern Brazil were not the same as those he used to see from the Mediterranean. The confusing thing is that once the continent was named America in the 16th century and Latin America was so named in the

19th century, it was as if those names had always existed. “America” was never a continent to be discovered but an invention forged in the process of European colonial history and the consolidation and expansion of Western ideas and institutions. The stories of discovery did not belong to the inhabitants of Anahuac or Tawantinsuyu but to the Europeans. It took 450 years for a transformation in the geography of knowledge to take place, and what Europe saw as a “discovery” came to be seen as an invention.

(2007)

i.

For some time now, at the École Lacanienne de Psychanalyse, of the

and which involved the spiritual conquest of native peoples and those brought over in slavery. Little is said about spiritual coloniality, which leaves in the background a dimension without which little could have been “conquered”.[4]

I would like to paraphrase Donna Haraway and her “we have never been human” to say: “we have never been Catholic”.

Jean Allouch, who in turn shakes hands with Foucault, acknowledged that psychoanalysis is a spiritual exercise. Of course, up to that point, in the response to Foucault in *Psychoanalysis is a Spiritual Exercise* (Allouch, 2007), it was about the spirituality of the philosophical schools of antiquity. Gradually, however, Lacan’s Catholic influence became more and more evident, something of which he himself seemed to be more than aware, and which led him to practise a marking as much as a constant unmarking of those theological presuppositions that were essential to the Western subjective constitution.

Jacques Lacan seemed to walk on that edge, as suggested by several indications, more recently confirmed by Sara Vasallo (2015). Producing a “viable atheist” at the end of an analysis will be for some a logical necessity if not an ideal (we already know that one puts them out the door and they return through the window). A viable atheist, or what amounts to the same thing, “someone who does not contradict himself at every turn”, Lacan would say, a full-time atheist, I ask not without irony. But is there only one way of the spiritual? Does the Catholic hegemony, colonial in these parts, annul other spiritualities, pre-existing or the result of the slave trade in the misnamed Latin America? This is a hegemony which, on the other hand, we have known for some time now is more than shaky; the Protestant churches have thousands of followers and exorbitant amounts of money, but African, Afro-Brazilian, Afro-Cuban, etc., spirituality also brings together thousands more, and in Mesoamerica and South America. From a greater awareness, indigenous spiritualities, far from dying out, are making a comeback, or simply gaining visibility, since they never disappeared.

Or would this, paradoxically, reinforce it in its pretended colonial, universalising hegemony? Does talk of a great Other, of divine omnipotence, of the jouissance of the Other, account for these other ways of being in relation to the divine? Even the very notion of the divine, of spirit, of Grace, should perhaps be revisited in the light of other spiritualities, hitherto the object of ignorance, of inadvertence.

The same Jean Allouch – albeit in a different sense – in the introduction to *The Sex of the Master* (2009) warns that it is no longer possible to speak of "true religion" in relation to the Catholic religion:

> Let us therefore consult the appropriate person, in this case Cardinal J. Ratzinger. . . . What is his answer to the question put to him: "2000 years after what?" As a theologian, and not only as a pastor, he evokes the only possible starting point for his answer, namely the victory of Christianity over Roman paganism, which is the victory of Christianity over Roman Catholicism.
>
> Nietzsche revolted against this victory in the most precious manner, for he pointed out that the monotheistic God who had achieved it was an imaginary figure. To what, then, was this victory due? The Cardinal's answer: to the fact that Christianity was a rational knowledge. This is what was meant by the expression religio vera (which was taken for an opinion of Lacan's when it was only a quotation of the most usual kind). More explicitly: The force that transformed Christianity into a world religion consisted in the synthesis between reason, faith and life. But as the cardinal theologian honestly ascertains, this synthesis no longer holds, reason is no longer recognised as being present in the doctrine of faith, since on the contrary, according to the Buddha's parable of the Hindu king, the blind men and the elephant, reason in its modern version indicates that there can only be opinions about God. A king in northern India had one day gathered all the blind inhabitants of the city in one place. Then he made an elephant pass in front of those present. He let some touch the head saying, "This is an elephant." Others could touch the ear or the tusk, the trunk, the leg, the haunches, the tail hairs. The king asked each one: "What is an elephant like?" And they answered according to the part they had touched: "It is like a plaited grey hair . . . it is like a pot . . . it is like the handle of a plough . . . it is like a silo . . . it is like a pillar . . .". Whereupon they began to argue and shouting "The elephant is this, the elephant is that" they threw themselves upon each other and beat each other with their fists to the amusement of the king. Let it be thus recorded: there is henceforth no "true religion" in the West.

In *Prisoners of the Great Other. La injerencia divina i*, Jean Allouch (2013) recognises the validity – the heuristic value, as he calls it – of Francois Jullien's journey through Chinese thought and culture in order to delimit the Western in another way, but, he clarifies, this is not his aim:

> One immediately thinks of François Jullien's journey, his detour around China. The very clear otherness of Chinese thought allows him to question Western thought with new dividends, approaching it with unexpected questions, making it work in a different way than when he examines his own history. Several works now attest to this: the heuristic value of this back and forth is already established. However, I intend to invite my reader to something somewhat different.

For the journey considered here does not aspire to return to psychoanalysis with a view to raising new issues within it. *It is not an attempt to bring to light certain gaps or presuppositions in analytic knowledge, nor to finally bring to light certain previous, ignored, silent and yet operative decisions within knowledge.* On the contrary: the questions that are raised here about the established do not contain anything absolutely new, they are already present in the Freudian field, especially in Jacques Lacan. Nevertheless, they form the locus of an epistemological decision on my part which it is now time for me to make explicit.

What decision? A priori, I admit that these questions cannot be dealt with from the inside, solely by reading Freud, Lacan and a few others. In other words, I will provide myself with magnifying glasses, which will be called Marc-François Lacan, Bernard Sichère, Jean-Luc Marion, Jean-Christophe Bailly, Pier Paolo Pasolini, Romeo Castellucci . . .

The contemporary works that will function as so many magnifying glasses can be classified into three categories that constitute different relationships with Christianity.

i. The first category is notoriously Christian; it is devoted either to recovering Lacan (Marc-François Lacan), or to reviving the God whose death was announced by Nietzsche and some others (Bernard Sichère, Jean-Luc Marion). Taken as a whole, the first category poses to analysis the crucial question of the call of the Other.
ii. A second category, on the contrary, assumes the decision to put an end to the dead god (Jean-Christophe Bailly) and the question will then be to know at what price it would be possible, if such a price is acceptable for analysis, but also if it is the right one for the death of God or of the gods.
iii. The third category (Pasolini, to whom one could add Lacan and, very recently, Castellucci) is aware that Christianity has not said its last word, so he maintains a tense relationship with Christianity. As a child, Lacan suckled on Christianity, a few years later his paternal grandfather taught him to curse God, while his death raised the question of a possibly Catholic funeral. Those who think, albeit too hastily, of a Christian Lacan as distinct from a Jewish Freud are therefore not talking plain stupidity. Many psychoanalysts come from there, and their silence about Christianity, even their Christianity, is striking, just as the mediation by which some transfer a most traditional Jewish morality to analysis without ever saying where they get what they present as knowledge arising from psychoanalytic experience is striking. The same was not true of Lacan, or Pasolini, or Castellucci, who obviously did not fail to deal with Christianity.

(Allouch)

Epistemic honesty should be emphasised when it comes to putting on the table the instruments, the magnifying glasses with which to operate, on the understanding that these will in turn be the limits and the scope of the work to be done. It is perhaps less comparable to equate *God and the gods* in an act of erasure of the differences that I do not believe to be appropriate. Erasure that reproduces the colonising sweep of the conquest of the spirits.[5]

The observation of the Christian and the Jewish operating in psychoanalysis is not striking, but neither should it be naturalised, since it has exclusionary effects and consequences for other spiritualities which, without operating in the doctrinal field, do so in the lives of people who are eventually analysed or intend to be analysed. And contrary to the manifest design of *Prisoners of the Big Other*, here it will be a matter of "making certain spiritualities appear".

> gaps or presuppositions of analytical knowledge, . . . to finally update certain previous decisions, ignored, silent and yet operative within knowledge.

ii.

"Why Olodumare is not God" will be an attempt to answer the question of what makes a supposed creator God or not and what effects the fact of monotheism or polytheism, of omnipotence or of multiplicity and division of powers, of a generated or degenerated deity, etc., has on this divine constitution. What are the consequences for the subjects of the fact that "sacred" entities not only do not hide their imperfections, their faults, but that these are the sign, the reason for their potency, for their power?

The "Axé", in order to introduce us to another language without which no spirituality seems to be sustainable. To do so, we will take *Candomblé* – a religious expression of the African Yoruba diaspora – as well as its South American derivations resulting from syncretism and fusions with the indigenous and the Catholic.

Each head Orixá will mark his/her son/daughter with his/her characteristics. In this sort of second birth that is religious initiation, the legend will be re-actualised in an attempt to learn from it between repetition and overcoming, spiritual elevation. Olodumare is considered the head of the Yoruba pantheon that contains 1,700 divinities; he is Olofin-Orun, which means lord of the sky; he is also Olodumare, all-powerful and supreme. For the Yoruba of Nigeria, he is the discerner of hearts: "the one who sees the inside and outside of man", active in celestial and terrestrial affairs. Olodumare can do all things, is the facilitator of all who achieve any end. No one has ever seen him/her, but nevertheless Olodumare is regarded as the omnipotent one, a powerful and eternal rock, ever constant and reliable. He/she is impartial, controlling the destinies of humanity in his/her palm. It is widely accepted that the Orisha is the one who punishes humanity *when natural laws are broken*. However, Olodumare judges man in his innermost feelings, good character, and personality, because he/she knows the innermost desires, feelings, and thoughts.

Olodumare created the universe, appointed day and night, arranged the seasons, and fixed the destiny of men; when misfortune befalls a bad person, the Yoruba say that “he is under the eyelashes of Olodumare”. Death was also his creation, for in the beginning men did not die, they grew to an immense size, after which they were reduced to old and weak people because there were so many around them; men prayed to Olodumare, begging him to deliver them from a long life, and so the old men died.

However, despite or contrary to this supposed omnipotence and omnipresence of Olodumare, in the religious and life practice of the practitioners of Candomblé and Batuque, Olodumare is not referred to in this way, but mediated by the Orixas, mainly by the Orixas who rule the life of each person (head Orixa and adjuncts). And if we take into account that the Orixas represent forces of nature, human faults refer more to a breaking of laws considered natural, to the production of an imbalance of forces or energies, rather than to a moral fault that generates guilt.

There is a relationship with nature to be preserved insofar as one is part of that nature as living incarnations, “horses”, “matter” of the spirits or Orixas – forces of nature. I am not saying that there is no ethical or moral dimension at stake – even if this way of putting it is already the introduction of a Eurocentric notion – but that this ethical dimension, this ethos, will be a function of the community, of the collective, as much as of the relationship with nature in a productive indifferentiation. There is no human ethos separate from that which governs all beings.

The Orixas, in spite of their character as deities or “entities”, guides, etc., possess “weaknesses” or propensities that will characterise their children, constituting for them challenges to be overcome: Oxum is vain, Iemanjá vengeful, Xangó treacherous, Ogún impulsive, and these traits must be kept in check by the children of each Orixá, while constituting their potency.

The axé, the power of the Orixá, is the Achilles heel of the *hijx*. Of course, to speak of *vanity*, *vengefulness*, *betrayal*, is already a *translation* of what is not evident to be thought and experienced from this code of defects and virtues. The passage of languages contributes to the conquest and erasure. This also happens with notions such as spirit or God, Goddess, saint, witch, priest, etc.

A house of religion or Ile must then care for the balance of all these forces embodied in each son of Oryxa. Otherwise, internal war will ensue, and the house could be destroyed. There is a communal ethos which, besides being already part of the African tradition, had to be reinforced in the face of the torments of slavery. In fact, originally in Africa, each village was inhabited only by the children of one Oryxa, and in many cases they were at war with the people of another Oryxa. The slave trade and the diaspora forced them to make peace and even to unite ritually (today in a *batuque* or Oryxa feast, there are children of Bará, Ogún, Oiá, Oxum, Obaluaié, Oxalá, etc.) as a strategy of material and spiritual survival. Although stating it in this way again implies a division of material/spiritual, which does not operate in this way outside the West.[6]

One of the authors who questioned early on the relationship between Afrodiasporic spirituality and subjectivity was Rita Segato. Thus, in *The Brazilian Oedipus (*Segato, 2015), she highlights the *double negation* of gender and race of the figure of the Afro woman based on the observation of the mostly black presence in the figure of the nanny or milkmaid, for white children in Brazil; at the same time, she wonders about this erasure in psychoanalytic theorisations on the oedipal question.

For my part, I ask myself, what does this erasure or *erasure* – to use the term Lacan uses in the section I have chosen for this text – imply in terms of an other spirituality that is there, unknown? Inaugural erasure of a hygienist-racist modernity? And also, what does this ignorance imply in the production of subjects? From the reverse side of the racist device, Segato proposes to read the dissociation between the mother who gives birth and the mother who raises, that is, from the Yoruba mythology that embodies both figures in Yemanja and Oxum respectively:

> Iemanjá is described as a cold, hierarchical, distant and indifferent mother. Her mothering is conventional. Although tender in appearance, people say that her tenderness is more a consequence of her self-control and good manners than of a compassionate and tender heart – as opposed to the true affection of Oxum, the "adoptive mother". As a divinity associated with the sea, she is said to share its qualities. She is "treacherous" and "false", like the sea. Here we find evoked the historical betrayal of the Atlantic, when it brought slaves to the New World and definitively interposed its insurmountable distance from Africa.
>
> The element of "falsity" is a matter of the past, but one that links the coasts of the two continents in the present. The element of "falsehood" is explicitly attributed to the duplicity and unpredictability of the sea, whose surface hides underneath a turbulent depth that cannot be seen, making the emergence of storm surges unpredictable: "you see the surface, but you don't see the bottom", the cult people often say. In the snail oracle, Iemanjá, the "legitimate", biological and hieratic mother, "speaks" in two positions called Obedi and ossatunukó.
>
> (Segato, 2015)

The idea that the figure of the mother, from the division of tasks of childbirth-raising, resists idealisation in another way seems interesting. Likewise, Segato makes visible the pre-eminence of *order* over *justice* for the Yoruba people in the legend of Iemanja's illegitimate coronation of Xangó and not of Ogún, the son deserving of the throne. Segato's reading of this legend is political, or rather historical-political, of the survival of an enslaved and uprooted people:

> The political discourse of the myth is thus exposed. Its cryptic statement points to the lie that lies at the very foundation of the establishment and its laws. Although a latent ethical estrangement can be perceived, the intention of the mythical commentary is not to formulate an alternative moral status, but to produce a sociology, a hermeneutics proper to the social milieu. This pragmatic psychology – as I have called it elsewhere (Segato, 2015) – constitutes a survival manual under an alien and arbitrary regime.
>
> (Segato, 2015)

Rita Segato goes so far as to speak of an "Afro-Brazilian religious codex" (Segato, 2015). This "codex" – made of orality and not of images, although of an orality loaded with images – will function as "the civilising discourse of Afro-Brazilian religions and their historical project" (Segato, 2015).

.More recently, Tamy Ayouch (2018), a Moroccan psychoanalyst currently living and working in Paris, recounts her experience with Brazilian Candomblé in "From the binary to the multiple: gender subjectivities in Candomblé". Candomblé is understood as the site of a different configuration of gender relations. The author takes up the idea of P. De Aquino (2000), for whom the creation of the world does not rest on a union of opposites or on a cut of a full unity, but on a differentiation "without a prior differential position". Identity assignments are then mobile and are constituted in the ritual itself. The individual ceases to be "coincident with himself". The duality human-nonhuman, male-female, is fluidised, and sexual difference is called into question as ahistorical and universal. In this way, Candomblé would be inscribed as one more of the practices of hybridity alongside psychoanalysis that the author postulates along the lines of Homi Bhabha (1994).

iii.

Oyeronké Oyewumi (2017) in *The Invention of Women* points out that "Western theories and conceptual schemes have become so widespread that most researchers, including those of African origin, unquestionably use them". He will then write from "the understanding of Western dominance in African Studies":

> It came to seem so obvious to me, drawing an analogy with Michel Foucault's explanation of the history of sexuality, that the history of gender – that is, the history of what in academic discourse functions as a specific field of truth – had to be written first of all from the point of view of the history of discourses.

He adds:

> It will become essential to analyse "the ways in which Western assumptions of sexual difference are used to interpret Yorùbá society, thus creating a local gender system".
>
> 1- Gender categories are universal and timeless and have been present in every society at all times. The idea is often expressed in a biblical tone, as if to suggest that "in the beginning was gender". 2- Gender always stands out as a fundamental organising principle in all societies. Gender is everywhere in any given society. 3- There is an essential, universal category, "woman", characterised by the social uniformity of its members. 4- The subordination of women is universal. 5- The category "woman" is pre-cultural, immovable in historical time and cultural space and antithetical to another unalterable category – "man".

I argue that such assumptions derive from the fact that in Western societies physical bodies are always social bodies. Consequently, there is no real distinction between sex and gender, despite feminists' efforts to distinguish them. In the West, social categories have a long history of embodiment and thus engendering. According to anthropologist Shelly Errington, "Sex (with a capital S) is the gender system of the West". She continues:

> but Sex is not the only way to classify human bodies, nor is it the only way to signify sex. One could easily imagine different logics and cultural classifications for gender categories, different scenarios that in turn take into consideration the evidence offered by our bodies.

The Yorùbá case provides one such scenario. Moreover, it demonstrates that the human body does not need to be engendered to be constituted or seen on every occasion as an indication of social ranking. In pre-colonial Yorùbá society, body type was not the basis of social hierarchy: the social position of males and females did not depend on their anatomical distinction. Social order required a different cartography and not a gender map based on the assumption of biology as the foundation of social classification.

There will then be other ways of understanding people's social position, which will not be without consequences:

> Pre-colonial Yorùbá cultural logic did not use the human body as the basis of social rank (in Yorùbá society under no circumstances was a male inherently superior to a female by virtue of his body type), society was organised hierarchically, from enslaved people to those who governed. The rank of people depended first and foremost on seniority, which was usually defined by relative age. Another fundamental difference between Yorùbá and Western social categories is the highly situational nature of Yorùbá social identity. Before the sustained intrusion of Western categories, in Yorùbá society people's social positions were constantly changing in relation to those with whom they interacted; thus, social identity was relational rather than essentialist.
>
> (Oyewumi Oyeronkẹ́, 2017)

But it is not only the sex-gender system that reveals its non-universality here, but even a way of producing the world from a materiality that produces thought and subjectivity.

As the author explains, the reason why the body has been so relevant in the West is that the world is perceived first and foremost by sight. The differentiation of human bodies in terms of sex, skin colour and cranial size testify to the powers attributed to the "seer". Contemplation invites differentiation. Therefore, different approaches to the understanding of reality will imply epistemological differences between societies. Compared to Yorùbá society, the main focus of this paper, the body has an exaggerated relevance in the Western conceptualisation of society.

The term "worldview", which is used in the West to synthesise the cultural logic of a society, adequately expresses the Western prerogative of the visual dimension. But it is Eurocentric to use it to refer to cultures that may give priority to other senses. The qualifier "sense of the world" is a more open alternative to describe the worldviews of different cultural groups. Therefore, in this study "worldview" will be applied exclusively in describing the cultural sense of the West and "sense of the world" will be used in reference to Yorùbá society or other cultures that may privilege other senses or even a combination of them.

With regard to gender, a Western category, it will say:

> Gender is a dichotomous discourse on two social categories – male and female – in binary opposition and hierarchy. Given the above, my first point is that the common glossing of the Yorùbá categories obìnrin and ọkùnrin as "female/female" and "male/man", respectively, is a mistranslation. This error occurred because most Western intellectuals and Yorùbá intellectuals with Western influences failed to realise that in Yorùbá thought and practice these categories are neither in binary opposition nor hierarchical to each other.
>
> (Oyewumi, 2017)

Finally, the author points out that the different hierarchisation of the biological and the social between the West and the African Yoruba culture makes it impossible to simply transfer meaning.

iv.

Sara Vasallo (2015) says in "Jacques Lacan's Atheism":

> If it is indubitable that Lacan is an atheist, that does not mean that he is one. All his insistent irony against deists, atheists, Nietzscheans or freethinkers was always centred on arguing that "God" as a signifier refers to a Real that is impossible to eliminate. In other words, the atheist's denial: "God does not exist", does not cancel the contrary affirmation (God exists), indeed, it amounts to a denial, since a blind nucleus, linked to the "dead Father", subsists beyond the yes or no (the dead Father says nothing, he does not even know that he died, placing himself at a point of interruption of the message and signification). The question is, of course, to know what kind of atheism emerges from a logic where yes and no are superimposed without excluding each other. To answer this question it would be necessary to analyze step by step different moments of Lacan's teaching.
>
> The last phase, at a time when the relationship to the Father was formulated as: "To do without the father on condition of making use of him". In a similar way, one could also say of his atheism: "To do without religion on condition of

> making use of it". It will be said: make use of what in it? Of a Father who gives law and meaning, or rather, of a Name-of-the-Father (an expression already formulated in the Judeo-Christian religious narrative).

What Vasallo locates as a "rhetorical matrix" for Jacques Lacan's psychoanalysis, Christian theology, perhaps goes beyond that if we stop to think about the effects of this rhetoric. The Foucauldian – rather than the Lacanian – notion of discourse might shed light here on what causes this rhetoric. Real effects of discourses.

In any case, and provisionally assuming this thesis, is it not then necessary for each practitioner of psychoanalysis to do his or her own thing, that is, to question his or her relationship with the religious and/or spiritual matrixes that constitute him or her? And in the case of South American and Mesoamerican practitioners, does this not imply not ignoring other, non-Catholic spiritualities that are part of their culture, even if they are marginalised or silenced by genocide or other forms of erasure?

What does it mean to be part of a society that is proud of its European ancestry and of being a country "without Indians", while folklorising and appropriating Afro demonstrations, without this implying any real recognition? A country that claims to be atheist but closely follows the sayings of the Pope or the Archbishop and celebrates Holy Week under the pretext of tourism. A country in which other religious manifestations and non-Catholic spiritualities continue to grow, while the Catholic religion is irremediably decreasing.

v.

From the field of education (understood as an educational project), she begins by expressing her gratitude. The first step is to express gratitude to those who have offered their ancestral skills and practices. Gratitude is one of the values that political-poetic Luiz Rufino Rodrigues Junior (2018) in "Pedagogias das encruzilhadas" – an article that arises as a result of his PhD thesis in Education – proposes to produce "reconstructive wisdoms" based on inventions born in the frontiers and in the gaps that remain. His educational project proposes to "develop critiques and propose other paths with respect to the issues of racism, colonialism and education. The action here is to invoke and embody the powers of the Yoruba deity Exu transferred in the diaspora, to propose a Pedagogy of the Crossroads". (The crossroads is the realm of Exu, orixá of the limits and of the passage.)

It continues:

> Starting from the defence of the non-redemption of colonialism, questioning the continuity of its effects on the formation of a multiple and unfinished world, I read, here, the conceptual availability based on the crossroads of Exu, which emerges as a symbol of a different political/poetic/educational project. The pedagogy embodied by the powers of the orixá weaves a balance of multiple concepts that confront the arrogance and primacy of forms constructed by colonial logic. In this way, rather than confronting the limits of the dominant reason, the proposal launched for now points to other paths: from inventions born on the

> frontiers and in the gaps that remain, they are reconstructive wisdoms of the beings who, in the invention of the New World, were presented to the politics of subordination, imprisonment and death of race/racism.

There is in Rufino Rodriguez a provocative political wager that involves a spiritual and subjective hacking of the colonial matrix of education and the state.

vi.

Roberto Strongman (2019), in *Queering Black Atlantics religions. Transcorporeality in Candomble, santeria and Voudou*, Strongman claims to have learned from his research. It is interesting to note that in these spiritualities values are themselves and at the same time energy, power, and potency, *axé*. Strongman centres his work around the notion of transcorporeality: Afrodiasporic culture's distinctive representation of the human psyche as multiple, removable, and external to the body, which functions as a receptacle. And to give some representation of this he uses the cashew nut:

> a tropical fruit that is largely unknown in Europe and North America because the fragility of its skin prevents export. However, this emblematic and queer fruit, arising from the flora of the geographical and climatic region covered in this book, is widely cultivated and consumed on both sides of the black Atlantic by humans and gods, as it is a favourite offering of the orishas Changó and Oshún.
>
> The cashew pear (*P. pomme de cajou*, Sp. Marañón, Pg. Caju, Kreyòl pomkajou, also known by the taxonomic name Anacardium occidentale) allows us to easily see how the transcorporeal conceptualisation of the body is sustained. The core of the self, not within the flesh of the fruit, but on the outside . . . that speaks of the externality, flight, and Ashé-potency of the transcorporeal spirit.
>
> . . . This experience in which the self or soul: . . . exists in an external orientation vis-à-vis the physical body, enables the regeneration of the bodies of the initiates.
>
> Mounted by deities of a gender other than their own during the ritual ecstasy of trance possession . . . transcendental moments in which the blending of the human and the divine produces subjectivities whose gender is not dictated by biological sex. In doing so, he demonstrates that, while transcorporeality has its roots in the religious practice of trance possession, its effects extend into people's everyday lives.

vii.

From France, Cherif Zahar Farah, Irrera Orazio, Kisuki:

> The aim of the project is to create non-European archives, while trying to free oneself from the concepts and distinctions imposed by the colonial cartography

of philosophy and, consequently, to question the formation of categories. The aim of the project is to explore the canonical "European/Western philosophy" and to measure the limits of distinctions such as Europe/non-Europe, West/non-West.

To wrest philosophy from a geography which, even today, causes it to confuse the limits of its "territory" with the borders, real or imagined, of the West: such is, in its most general and even negative expression, the programme pursued by several members of our department who share the requirement of reciprocal empowerment between the critical re-reading of Western philosophical traditions and their decentralisation, which implies the revision of their metaphysical and anthropological assumptions, no less than the dominant historiographies of philosophy. This seminar aims to bring together forces and confront heterogeneous approaches, closely associating students with this enterprise to which we would like to lend a dimension that is not only descriptive but also prescriptive in terms of philosophical teaching and research in France.

Exploring the non-European archives of philosophy, a task inseparable from its (re)construction, has three meanings here. First, it implies re-examining the canon of the discipline, its subjects, authors and reference texts, and measuring the effects generated by its confrontation with a range of knowledge and counter-knowledge, produced outside Europe, whether they have given themselves the name of philosophy or not. The second is to reconsider its objects by analysing the way in which the "encounter" between Europe and non-European worlds, under the dominant sign of violence (slavery, colonial, imperialist) but also of resistance, contributed to shape a whole set of more or less classical philosophical problems, which the singular representations made seemingly foreign to these same experiences of violence and resistance. Thirdly, it will seek to question the very enterprise itself.

viii.

To conclude, for now, I would like to revisit some of the epistemic considerations that Valentin-Yves sip Mudimbe (1988) made in his now canonical *The Invention of Africa. Gnosis, philosophy and the order of knowledge*. He begins his book with epistemic considerations:

> Strictly speaking, the notion of African philosophy refers to the contributions of Africans practising philosophy within the framework of the discipline and its historical tradition. It is only metaphorically or, at best, from a historicist perspective, that the notion of philosophy can be extended to traditional African systems of thought, considering them as dynamic processes in which concrete experiences are integrated into an order of concepts and concepts of discourses (Mudimbe, 1988).
>
> So I preferred to speak of African gnosis. J. Fabian used the notion of gnosis in his analysis of a charismatic movement (Mudimbe, 1988).

In this book, the broader framework seems to be more appropriate for the set of problems addressed, all based on a preliminary question: to what extent can one speak of African knowledge and in what sense? Etymologically, the term *gnosis* is related to gnosko, which in ancient Greek means "to know".

> Specifically, *gnosis* means the search for knowledge, research, methods of knowledge, investigation and even familiarisation with someone. Often, the word is used in a more specialised sense, that of a higher, esoteric knowledge, and therefore refers to structured, common and conventional knowledge, but under the control of specific procedures, with regard to both use for its transmission.
>
> Gnosis is therefore different from doxa or opinion and, on the other hand, cannot be confused with episteme, understood as both science and general intellectual configuration.
>
> The title is thus a methodological tool: it embraces the question of what African philosophy is and what it is not, and also orients the debate in another direction, focusing on the conditions of possibility of philosophy as part of a broader body of knowledge about Africa called "Africanism".
>
> I use this central notion of conditions of positionality in a recent tradition, through which Michel Foucault was able, for example, to define his own intellectual ambition in terms of its dependence on the changes that Jean Hyppolite had introduced into Hegelian philosophy (Foucault, 1994: 74–82). What the notion of conditions of possibility indicates is that discourses not only have sociohistorical origins, but also depend on epistemological contexts.

Mudimbe thus sets himself the ambitious goal of producing a kind of "archaeology of African gnosis", of the African mode of knowledge. Like Oyeronké Oyewumi, he is aware of the fact that "until now, both Western interpreters and African analysts have used categories and conceptual systems that depend on a Western epistemological order". Just as one speaks from a certain position or place of enunciation, one also thinks and produces knowledge from a certain place. In this sense, Mudimbe proposes the notion of a "non-African epistemological locus". This will then be an *analysis of discourses* on Africa, which is paradoxically a very Western way of trying to dissociate oneself from the Western episteme.

An interesting element in this author's analysis is what he calls *marginal space* or *in-between space*, a space *between* the effects of the colonisation of Africa, where the tension between the pre-tension of modernisation and "an impoverished image of a mythical past" remains unresolved.

As proof enough . . . or so the saying goes, I invite you to think about the gesture of turning ritual, religious objects into art – African art, one might say. And this, which in the eyes of Pierre Bourdieu – if it were given in an inverted way – would be a categorical error, supposes a mode of colonial appropriation-expropriation that operates on a different spirituality, making it become "a mysterious diversity of the Same" or "a negative category of the Same", according to Mudimbe's two felicitous expressions.

By way of non-conclusion

And in order not to keep on finding only confirmations of the same thing – variants or diversities – or rather, to bet on making room for something really other – although the one and the other are still part of the fatal binarism of language – I propose to assent to the existence of other spiritualities that also operate as a matrix of subjectivities, and that it is necessary not to ignore from a psychoanalysis that pretends to be *non-colonial* . . . if such a thing is possible.

Non-existence of the subject, transcorporeality, and other entanglements

In a previous work,[7] I tried to problematise the idea that psychoanalysis can only accommodate a subject constituted on the basis of the Cartesian subject, produced in the subjective matrix of Catholic spirituality. Among other reasons, because in the South America in which I live and practice psychoanalysis, this would imply ignoring other ways of producing subjects as well as other spiritualities and ways of conceiving both the so-called social bond and the social itself.

The contemporary crisis of the notion of *kinship*, through writings such as those of Marilyn Strathern, Donna Haraway, Viveiros de Castro, and others, opens up the possibility of other rivals, for example along the lines of what Marshall Sahlins (2011) has called "mutuality of being".

> Generally speaking, kin are people who belong to each other, who are part of each other, who are co-present in each other, whose lives are linked and interdependent.

Kinship – perhaps the plural is appropriate – would be more on the side of the exchange of gifts and magic, bringing beings and things into relationship. And it is perhaps in the abandonment of what Oyeronké Oyewumí (2017) in *The Invention of Women*, calls *bio-logic*, that some of this can be understood.

Clara Flaksman (2018) from the University of Rio de Janeiro stated:

> The person in candomblé is a set of his relationships (his *entanglements*) whose equilibrium and completeness are always ephemeral. The person is formed diachronically, but its completeness is always synchronic – it is completed in a moment and then decompleted later. To have *entanglement* is to be part of something, to have a part of it, that is to establish a communion of substances with it, it is to possess a relationship of kinship, it is to carry a little of the other. There are boundaries between people, orixás, entities and things that are fluid, and that can be crossed with the right *technology*.
>
> (Translation and italics are mine)

Of course, as I understand it, some terms such as completeness, personhood, etc. would have to be problematised, but the idea that something of the being-in-fault is constituted in its entanglements seems interesting.[8] The idea of entanglements is also present in Donna Haraway (2019a), although it should be clarified that the *entanglement* in Candomblé is specific in relation to Orixas and entities of Yoruba cosmopolitics. Says Haraway:

> Rooted in unities and relations, especially competitive relations, the sciences of modern synthesis – population genetics, for example – have serious problems with four key biological domains: embryology and development, symbiosis and *collaborative entanglements* of holobionts and holobiomes, the vast configuration of microbial worlds, and the exuberant bio-behaviours and inter/intraactions of bugs. Approaches attuned to *"becoming-with-multi-species"* best help us to pursue the problem on terra.
>
> (Italics are mine)

On the other hand, Flaksman's final reference to technology – "borders that are fluid and can be crossed with the appropriate technology" – makes me think of a re-signification of the Foucauldian notion of *technologies of the self.* Resignified given that here the self is not embodied (with all the mess that flesh entails for Catholic spirituality) in a being but in a multiple entanglement. Derivations that involve the self from kinship and even make it become insufficient: it is no longer a relationality of beings that exist separately, but rather in agency, beings that are composed mutually in hybrid, symbiogenetic, interspecies becomings.

For reasons of my personal history, I was introduced to the ritual practice of the so-called Afroumbandist religions, of Yoruba roots, which, through syncretism, keep alive African traditions and cosmogonies. It is from there that it is quite clear to me that, if, as Jean Allouch and others suggest, spirituality is the matrix of subjectivation of subjects, when dealing with spiritualities that are not centred on the subject and/or that do not even possess the very idea of the subject, we are faced with another reality that should not be ignored. There are researchers, mainly from the anthropological field (Goldman, 1985), who are led to think of a complexification of the notion of personhood constituted in a ritual way and in the hybridisation with non-human entities, in a long initiatory process. However, if any of this carries a subjective truth, the very notion of personhood does not seem to hold much water.

Perhaps the assumption of a soul and a person is as racist as the question about the existence of a soul that the settlers of the American territory asked themselves. I find it appalling to deprive someone of a soul insofar as the individual soul is accorded the very status of the human, which in turn presupposes speciesist superiority over those who do not possess it. But what if the individual soul was not so highly valued? What if the notion of the individual and the person did not find an echo in a strongly transpersonal, transgeneric, trans-species, transcorporeal spiritual matrix either (Strongman, 2019)?

This questioning has a long history, as Virginia Fons (2005) rightly points out:

> The debate on the concept of personhood in anthropology arose as early as the 1940s, from Mauss's 1938 article entitled "Une catégorie de l'esprit humain: la notion de personne et celle de 'moi'". In the same vein, the 1947 publication by Leenhardt also appeared
>
> In the same vein, the 1947 publication by Leenhardt also appeared the concept of personhood in Melanesia entitled: *Do Kamo: Personhood and Myth in the Melanesian World.* This whole debate raised the centrality of the notion of personhood in the framework of any anthropological research. In other words, the argument was that any study of a society must consider what is meant by "personhood", how it is formed, what its components are, how they relate to each other and to the environment, and many other questions.

As early as 1971, he recalled:

> A colloquium on the concept of the person in Africa sought to bring together various specialists on this subject and on the African context, many of them disciples of Mauss. The Colloquium resulted in proceedings published under the title *La notion de personne en Afrique noire* (1993 [1973]). Most of the articles are contributions on the subject in the different cultures studied by the authors.

This colloquium was held in Paris as part of the international colloquia of the National Centre for Social Research, and its proceedings have been collected by G. Dieterleng (1993). Fons highlights the work of Roger Bastide and L. V. Thomas (1993):

> which set out two basic concepts for understanding the notion of personhood in Africa: that of unity and that of plurality. Although both concepts seem contradictory, they are not at all, as we will see in this article. To summarise Bastide's contribution (1993 [1973]), in Africa, populations have a notion of personhood but no clear concept of their individuality. According to this author, there are two anti-principles of individuality: the plurality of the constituent elements of the personality and the fusion of the person in his environment, in his otherness. In other words, it is not conceived as divisible or autonomous, as a being radically distinct from the things that surround it. It is not endowed with borders or boundaries. It is not outside the group. It is not a distinct member, although it may have a great deal of strength (the case of the chief, the warrior, the exceptional hunter or the sorcerer).
>
> (in Fons, 2005)

On the other hand, says Fons:

> Thomas's article (1993 [1973]) focuses more on the concept of *plurality*, since the person is the result of different forces coming together. At its core are different instances, invisible or not, vital or auxiliary, variable or immutable.

> Particularly interesting is his attempt to make the notion of the person more comprehensible, which should include that which is given or innate and inherited, acquired from the environment or from individual promotion, temporarily or definitively lost, desired or refused. Without all this being incompatible with awareness, with all kinds of substitutions or partial changes and definitive or provisional metamorphoses. This pluralism definitively breaks with a monolithic and static concept of the person and turns it into a kind of prism that contemplates a variety of possibilities. In other words, it leads us to introduce the idea of mutability or variability of the person throughout life and after death. (1993 [1973]).

E. Ortigues circumscribed his paper in relation to psychoanalysis: *La teoría de la personalidad en psicoanálisis y en etnología (Personality theory in psychoanalysis and ethnology)*. And even if in Lacanian psychoanalysis the notion of personality – in exception of Lacan's thesis ([1932] 2006a): *Of paranoid psychosis in its relations to personality* – was abandoned, it would nevertheless be interesting to revisit the subject-personality relationship,[9] which in principle seem to oppose each other.

Much more recently, Roberto Strongman, from Duke University, has come up with the notion of "transcorporeality", the power of which is more than interesting: "What would characterise this distinctive representation of Afrodiasporic culture is a notion of the human psyche as multiple, removable, and external to the body, which functions as a receptacle" (Strongman, 2019).

Today, as I intend to refine some notions, I would call this subjective production neither psyche nor human.

> a tropical fruit that is largely unknown in Europe and North America because the fragility of its skin prevents export. However, this emblematic and queer fruit, arising from the flora of the geographical and climatic region covered in this book, is widely cultivated and consumed on both sides of the black Atlantic by humans and gods, as it is a favourite offering of the orishas Changó and Oshún. The cashew pear (*P. pomme de cajou*, Sp. Marañón, Pg. Caju, Kreyòl pomkajou, also known by the taxonomic name Anacardium occidentum, Pg. taxonomical name Anacardium occidentale)[10] allows us to makes it easy to see how the transcorporeal conceptualisation of the body is sustained. The core of the self, not within the flesh of the fruit, but on the outside . . . that speaks of the externality, flight, and Ashé-power of the transcorporeal spirit.

And he adds:

> This experience in which the self or soul: exists in an external orientation vis-à-vis the physical body, allows for the regeneration of the bodies of the initiates. Mounted by deities of a gender different from their own during the ritual ecstasy of trance possession . . . transcendental moments in which the blending of the human and the divine produces subjectivities, whose gender is not dictated by

> biological sex. In doing so, he demonstrates that, while transcorporeality is rooted in the religious practice of trance possession, its effects extend into the everyday lives of the participants and observers of these religions and become a major feature of almost every aspect of Afrodiasporic cultural production.
>
> (Strongman, 2019)

As you will see, paradoxically,

> In Uruguay and, I suppose, in neighbouring countries, we also know it as cashew nuts. The possession or trance – "occupation" they will say in Candomblé and Batuque – of the initiate makes his/her body-matter the "horse" that the deity or Orixá rides. And in being occupied, the initiate's self will be vacated, making room for another, hybrid being or subjectivity, neither fully human nor divine. And if the Orixas are forces of non-human nature – to put it in western terms – this subjective becoming in trance will erase the boundaries initiated with the *borí* and the preparations in Orixá, the second birth of the child of religion.

Notions such as identity, proper name, and sexual-generic assignment deserve to be revisited then, in the light of this other form of subjectivation.

Thamy Ayouch (2020), who does not hesitate to situate psychoanalysis as a hybrid practice, argues that in Candomblé, identity assignments are mobile and are constituted in the ritual itself. The individual ceases to be "coincident with himself". The human-non-human, male-female duality is fluidised, calling into question sexual difference as ahistorical and universal. This non-coincidence with oneself of the Candomblé practitioner should not, I believe, be equated with the non-coincidence resulting from the subjective division, as we understand it in psychoanalysis. Perhaps it is a question of other subjective divisions and compositions as well as other constitutive agencies.

On the other hand, let us recall what Lacan (1967) said in *Brief Discourse to Psychiatrists* about the declaration of sex, in a Spinozian key:

> The experience of analysis is nothing other than the realisation of what is this function, as such, of the subject. It turns out that this opens up to a certain effect which shows us that in what is primarily concerned with this function of the signifier, there is a predominant difficulty, a flaw, a hole, a lack, of this signifying operation, which is very precisely linked to the confession, the articulation of the subject insofar as it is affected by a sex.

It seems quite obvious that the subject is a sexed subject. However, in this way of putting it, Lacan reveals the inconsistency of that which will be nothing more or less than an *affectation*; something with which the subject is made up. (In)signifying consistency which makes the western sex-gender system admit only two positions: male-female, man-woman.

In the same lecture, Lacan will speak of the *symbolic concealment* that makes the consistency of the sexual, its writing, impossible. The organ of copulation – as he calls it – is missing at this level and will be sought in the real as the penis. The inexistence of sexual relation seems to precipitate the reification of sexual difference. It is then a question of "the confession of the subject as affected by a sex", Lacan will say on this occasion; and I cannot fail to point out the pertinence of the term *confession*, even, and with all the more reason, if the use of this term were ironic.

Finally, all this roundabout to say that although the West has made sexual difference an indispensable subjective condition, it is only sustained on the signifying plane, despite the intentions of its reification. Or as Paul B. Preciado (2019b) stated, as a scientific religion or visual political regime, political epistemology. So, what are the consequences for the exercise of analysis of someone whose subjective matrix has taken place – at least in part – in another spiritual matrix?

They'll tell me that if someone goes to an analyst, he/she participates in something of the agreement that locates in psychoanalysis a place where something of their being might come to be concerned. Undoubtedly, the most probable thing – and in fact I can attest to this (if I may use the expression, ironic in this context) – is that we find ourselves with someone who participates in at least two matrices of subjectivation, in a complete hybridisation, not to be reduced; which, if we do, would constitute a form of violence and mastery of the master. Lacan was already aware of some of this. Thus, on one occasion when he receives people from the Upper Togo he will say:

> their unconscious functioned according to the good rules of the Oedipus. It was the unconscious that had been sold to them along with the laws of colonisation. . . . Their unconscious was not that of their childhood memories – this was palpable – but their childhood was lived retroactively with our familiar categories.
>
> (Lacan [1969–1970], 1992)

It is comforting to identify in Lacan something of a warning about the spiritual coloniality that must not be asserted in analytic practice. Subject, subjectivity, person, soul, spirit, in-consciousness, and a long list of other terms are all curled up to be no longer deconstructed but perhaps decolonised, de-universalised, situated, restated, rediscovered, and invented in a practice that does not deny the material imprints – which include the materiality of language – colonial and subjective-political of which we are the effect.

Notes

1 Although it is in bad taste to explain a title, like explaining a joke, it seems to me necessary to say that other versions than the father alludes to the homophonic play in French between perversion and père-version, as a version to (or of? I always read it as "of")

the father, introduced by Jacques Lacan (1974–75) with regard to this term in his seminar *rsi*.

2 This magical-religious dimension will be taken up both by the *Tiqqun* collective and by various authors, including Isabelle Stengers and Giorgio Agamben. Previously, Max Weber and Walter Benjamin had made their contributions in this regard.

3 However, as Oyéronke Oyéwúmí (2017) points out, nothing makes the sex of Olodumare evident – if this were not already an absurd anthropomorphisation of this greater Yoruba entity.

4 Even the notion of the coloniality of being, initially proposed by Walter Mignolo (2007), points more to the relation of being to language while ignoring the spiritual dimension.

5 I play here with the "spiritualist" dimension of the term "spirit".

6 In this sense, Silvia Rivera Cusicanqui (2018), in the presentation in Montevideo of his book *Un mundo Ch'ixi es posible*, proposes to characterise American spiritualities as "materialistic spiritualities", which, far from being an oxymoron, opens up possibilities for a greater understanding of the past, but which links the coasts of the two continents in the present.

7 Why Olodumare is not God, p. 182.

8 Perhaps in this approach some of this constitutive lack is resolved, albeit only in a transitory way.

9 In *The Sinthome*, Lacan ([1975] 2006) will say that it is not a question of relations between paranoia and personality, but that both are one and the same thing.

10 In Uruguay, and I suppose in neighbouring countries, it is also known as cashew nut.

Chapter 4

Lituras

Herman Melville: Furrowing loves, about *Billy Bud, Sailor*[1]

I know that this text has something of the cathartic, of the alluvial, of the only half-thought, though not so much; of that which does not want a punctuation that coheres, controls, or inhibits the disparted or even delirious production, if that is the case. I assume the risks, in the understanding that I find myself among companions of uncertainty, among seekers, adventurers, and not among colonisers of some truth or knowledge that pretends to know itself. I take the licence – poetic or not, I will not be the one to say so – to play with terms that today concern and challenge me: south, to love, loves, not loves, to walk, to sail, to cross, seas, and I could go on in an excess, an excess of resonances.

For someone like me who, in addition to analytical practice, is involved in writing, the fact of referring to a writer, bridging gulfs, to a peer, and taking him as a discursive excuse to say something that perhaps I could not say without his saying it, appears to me as something similar to sailing rough seas of ideas, of shared experience, of what I will make him say in an act of reading impossible to carry out without some hermeneutic, interpretative violence. I recognize myself in this partiality, in this bias, and in others; they seem to me, at least, to be ethical safeguards of an ethics that is always singular, provisional and that must be reviewed each time.

If we add to this the vicissitudes of an eroticism that insists on calling itself *gay* against the grain of a more politically correct affiliation with a certain universalising drift of the queer,[2] we can see that the gamble is not without risk. To read something of this eroticism and its subjective, subversive affects in someone who did not produce an overtly gay or homosexual literature, as he might – if we adhere to the Foucauldian idea of a precise historical dating of the notion of homosexuality, of its invention subsequent to or concomitant with the period of Melville's writing – might make us believe that we have been lost at sea, to continue with the marine allegory.

However, this may not be the case. In fact, it is fair to say that we have been preceded by several author-readers who have interviewed, intuited, and felt called upon by this reading bias. Incidentally, the excellent work by Rodrigo Andrés (2006), from the University of Valencia: *Herman Melville, poder y amor entre*

DOI: 10.4324/9781003710295-4

hombres, problematises this issue of what to call love between beings of the same sex before the nomination "homosexual".

Thus, those who resort to Greek pederasty to account for something homoerotic believe they are alluding to an erotic figure, or worse, to a figure of love and not to a mode of relationship oriented towards the education of the young men of the Athenian aristocracy – this is my position. A political relationship of power of moral and military transmission but not a figure of love between men. Love, homoeroticism which, however, coexisted all the time, although less visible with the relationship between *erastés* and *eromenos*.

On the other hand, something of the vicissitudes of Melville's life, of his suffering the incomprehension and outright rejection of his contemporaries, is not lost on me. I don't know if everyone knows, but after *Moby Dick* was published there was a dense silence in response, and Melville had a hard enough time with this. That he was suspected of insanity by those closest to him (he was said to be mad all the time), his silence for dozens of years in seclusion in an office, make him in my eyes almost a creature of his own invention, someone to be taken care of with great delicacy, and for this very reason they make him lovable.

The presence of Nathaniel Hawthorne, a neighbouring writer and reader of early versions of his writings (to whom Melville would dedicate *Moby Dick*) is a presence that brings only some relief, as Hawthorne was very ambivalent about Melville.

If, as Cuauhtémoc Medina (2010) points out, "the south is not a region, it is a currency of invention, deviation and resistance", it seems to me that the particular treatment of the erotic-political bond between men, which questions power and its reasons, can or could be thought of as a southern position. I am interested in rethinking the destabilising potential of love between men, politically destabilising, insofar as rivalry, submission, or a fight to the death is expected of them, or between them, but never love,[3] in any case, at most, a kind of chauvinism that is also called virile.[4] Even less so between those who are located in different social classes or power strata.

Something of this, it seems to me, claims an Alcibiades to a Socrates, who keeps to the terms expected by the pederastic codes. Precisely, something of this was intuited by Freud when he placed the homosexual bond at the basis of the viability of the social. Foucault saw something of this when he believed, albeit in a way that was as naïve as it was provocative, that the joy of a couple of gay lovers is more disturbing than their sexuality; and also when he thought that it was a question of creating new forms of relationship, new modalities of bonding.

The perspectives of Leo Bersani (1998) and David Halperin (2015) are more complex and would require further development. From the former, I am fundamentally interested in the location of the gay on the margins of the law, or at least in the promotion/invention of another law. From a morality of the minority, as Didier Eribon (2004) would want in Jean Genet's pistage? It is a question. Likewise, the idea of an *asocial relationality* of a rediscovery of the otherness of pure difference in fugitive contact, in the flirtation, in the gay transaction.

As for Halperin, the idea of a *sexual politics of truth* in which eroticism and truth are played together, inseparable, is an idea I would like to retain and do with. But none of this was on the horizon of what was thinkable for a nineteenth-century writer, which was no obstacle, however, to trying to pass something of another subjective positioning as much as to denouncing the discursive and real violence exercised on those who are placed in the position of subalterns, be they black, poor, subordinate, or rare, like a white whale or a beautiful, blond, sensitive sailor who believes in human rights.

The figure of Bartleby is perhaps one of the best known in Melville's literature. It has been the object of analysis – Deleuze's, particularly stirring – and is also a reference for authors such as Enrique Vila-Matas in his book *Bartleby y compañía*, which I suppose many have read, among others. It interests me that Vila-Matas (2015) speaks of "people who live and then stop living, but who deject the great enigma of writing that seems to be telling us that a voice says that life has no meaning but its deep timbre is the echo of that meaning". José Luis Pardo (2000) has also made fundamental contributions by emphasising the setting or maintenance in potency of every act in Bartleby's famous formula: "I would prefer not to". Something of a putting in suspension, which is potency in itself, creates and makes, gives rise to the emergence of something as yet undetermined.

Billy Budd, less well known, an unfinished story at the time of the author's death, appears to be condensing a multiplicity of features, ideas, minimal gestures, a word that hardly dares to be spoken and yet, like V., generates effects, resists. "It is the story of an innocence", an ethic and an aesthetic at the same time, of convictions that only manage to express themselves in stuttering, in hesitation (Billy Bud stutters). A not insignificant fact in relation to this work of Melville's old age is the death of his father-in-law, who was a judge, president of the Massachusetts Supreme Court, the first judge in the northern United States to have a runaway black slave returned to his master. This was Melville's father-in-law, on whom Melville will depend financially after the failures of his plays. In fact, some critics believe to see in the complex relationship with this father-in-law a relationship of domination and subjugation, albeit partial, which would allow the implementation of narrative strategies in which the location in a position of power character's point of view prevails (in many novels, this is what Melville does), which poses an ethical dilemma for the reader.

Billy Budd no longer has the vitalist, hopeful tone of the works of his youth. However, the subjective consequences of reading it can open up perspectives, sting and shatter ideas of justice, law, and established order. *Billy Budd, Sailor* is the story of the subversive power of beauty. It is also the story of a being who subverts a discursive logic that distributes places, ways of being and behaving, a logic of the virile, a logic of power that is based on submission to the word of the other, to a law beyond all justice.

At the end of the book, Captain Vere questions the impossible connection between law and justice. The incapacity for hatred in Billy Budd, or Baby Budd, as he will also be called, hinders his destruction. The character's hatred is expected, needed, a hatred that partly justifies the humiliations and injustices to which he is subjected. As Manuel Hernández (2013) says, "when it comes to the possibility or not of speaking (he refers to Spivac's work) the very core of psychoanalysis cannot remain intact", something that Melville shows once again, the last time, in this character who stutters in the face of the attempt at his subjective annulment.

Difficulty in articulating a word, a response, stammering, is less submission than a lucid awareness of the uselessness of any response. The act will then say and have its effects, not only negative. Melville will be lucidly aware that it is not a matter of telling the story of a hero without flaws, for it is precisely his imperfections, his particular ignorance, that Melville calls his incongruous strangeness, from which he will derive his transforming power. The beauty described without restraint or virile reticence sets the erotic tone of the story from the outset. I quote:

> She was young and despite her well-developed figure she looked even younger than she really was due to an adolescent expression that lingered on her still smooth, almost feminine face, in purity of natural colour but where, thanks to her travels by sea, the lily colour had almost completely disappeared and the pink had a hard time making itself visible in its blush through the tanning.

On her position on the ship: "she was analogous to a rustic beauty transplanted from the province and placed in competition with the aristocratic ladies of the court".

The gesture of comparing sailors on a British war frigate with ladies of a court is no small thing to me. Perhaps a double-meaning irony that crosses genres. He is compared to Hercules, to a thoroughbred horse, to Adam before the fall, to Apollo, to Achilles, to a barbarian; he is called a beautiful man, a beauty, and so on.

As Rodrigo Andrés points out, Billy Budd will alternatively be the noble savage, the blackness, the feminine, the pre-linguistic, the one who threatens the established order. He will also be the not-quite human in his ignorance of evil, like Claggart, master of arts, his antagonist, who is ignorant, or so he seems to pretend, of any logic other than that of Darwinian destruction that takes place in the depths of an apparently calm sea.

Billy Budd has, unsurprisingly, a tragic ending: the sailor is sentenced to death by hanging. This happens as an effect of a logic that will not cease to be questioned after Billy Budd kills Claggart with a blow when he is unable to defend himself verbally against false accusations. And he says: "if I could have used my tongue I wouldn't have hit him. I had to say something and I could only say it with a punch, God help me". Later it is said that this blow put a definitive brake on C.'s language, a question of loose languages and of brakes, of the possibility or impossibility of using one's own language. Can the subaltern speak? asks Spivac (2003). At the end of the novel, something of what must be silenced by the death of the handsome young sailor seems to want to reveal itself. It is about the feminine in the man that must be left out: "like a wailing woman who leads us astray with her pleas and appeals" with her other logic. I quote:

> The uniqueness of the matter stirs your hearts, says the captain of the ship, mine too is moved. But let not warm hearts betray heads that should be cool. The heart of which we speak is the feminine in man, and however hard it may be, it must be left out.
>
> (Melville)

While there is something of the mystified in this character, which has something of the saint, the Christ, the sacrificial, the angel, *the divine inertia* that Melville talks about in *Moby Dick*, it seems to me that this does not detract from the stirring and corrosive potential of this figure.

It has been questioned whether Billy Budd is a character or not. Rather, I think he should be seen not as a type, a character, but as a subjective position, another way of being in the world. It is not because he is unaware of his origin, his date of birth – the same is true of Bartleby, who lacks any biography – that his family novel can be woven and unwoven by him, by others, by us. This original mystery relaunches the question of identity, of what is bastard in each of us, of the wrongness of all filiation. In short, for the unfinished possibility of remaking ourselves and the collectives that adopt and adopt us.

Jean Genet: Life as a pretext, or becoming a shadow of the shadow

i. A question of method

I have long believed that, at least in psychoanalysis, if there is an ethic of writing, it has to do with writing about that by which one is touched, taken, concerned, pierced, wounded, or however you prefer. That is to say, at the greatest possible distance from all egoic pretensions of domination, of mastery, of knowledge; even in the knowledge that all discourse has a claim to dominance and owes claims to the discourse of the master, as Lacan (1997) reminds us in *The Reverse of Psychoanalysis*. Secondly, something of the fragmentary has also been imposed on me for some time, and I submit to it. Something of a renunciation of the university claim to say everything, as if that were possible!

ii.

My first approach to the École Lacanienne de Psychanalyse was related – among other things that I think I know and many others that I don't – to the imposing gesture of welcoming *Gay and Lesbian Studies*. A gesture that I understand is not exhausted in itself but that it is convenient – for me and for others, or at least I hope so – to take to its limits, to unfold, to problematise, avoiding its prescriptive encryption.

It is in this understanding, and summoned-provoked by a Colloquium that dares to speak its name: *Erotics of domination*. I understand that Jean Genet still has something to tell us about it. To say Jean Genet is on the order of excess as the author of a vast and plural oeuvre. That is why I have decided to limit the approach to fragments, snippets of a writing that will touch on *Diary of the Thief* (1976), *Funeral Pomps* (1947), and some of *Querelle de Brest* (2003). I will leave out a lot. If, for example, we had taken the path of dramaturgy, the play *Les negres (The Blacks)* would perhaps have shortened the path, but I'm not sure if that would be convenient.

Warned by Genet himself and by Leo Bersani (1998), among others, of the ravages of any biographical pretension (Sartre's *Saint Genet* . . . would cost him years of suffering and silence), I decided to approach his writing from a position closer to taking notes, to bear witness to a testimony, to pass on something of an erotics of theft, betrayal, fear, submission, and abjection in an ascesis that will go from the act to the song, from life to the writing of life. Life as a pre-text and as an excuse to say-say-self. Writing as a profane spiritual exercise, towards a different *holiness* (I will try to show of what order), which necessarily passes through "Evil".

From *Diary of the Thief*:

> It is not a search for the past, but a work of art whose material-pretext is my life of yesteryear. It will be a present fixed with the help of the past, not the reverse. Let it be known then that the facts were what I say, but the interpretation I make of them is what I am and what I have made myself.
>
> (1976)

To make oneself one with the abject will be a form of *subversive fidelity* to the path-destiny that "has been given to one's fate". Neither fatalism nor resignation, let alone resentment – as Sartre would have it – but a doing something else with that which constitutes us: "a chain of emotions of which I do not know the first ones", he will say.

> To love a man is not just to let myself be disturbed by one of those details that I describe as nocturnal, because they establish in me a darkness in which I tremble (the hair, the eyes, a smile, the thumb, the thigh, the hair etc.) is to force these details to turn as much as they can into shadow, to *develop the shadow of the shadow, to* make it thicker, therefore, to multiply its dominion and to populate it with black.
>
> (1976)

In the midst of a struggle for political rights and social conquests, Jean Genet remains a thorn in the heart of the gay movement, and I would even say Queer, as a lucid eroder of any accommodation to forms of the social bond. At times more sceptical than many – Foucault included – not even betting on other modes of sociality. Didier Eribon (2004) rescues some of this in *A Morality of the Minority*. Leo Bersani will do his own in *Homos* (although the latter seems to want to place Genet in the ranks of a non-relational sociality, a non-subjective intimacy). Something of this unassimilability links Jean Genet to other damned such as the Lautreamont of *The Songs of Maldoror*, or Louis Ferdinand Céline, whom we still hesitate whether to celebrate or denigrate.

Homosexuality, pederasty – terms used by him – and robbery will be seen as twinned in an outside the law, outside a social and bourgeois us; at the same time, they will be other ways of moving towards beauty *in* and *through* the act. An act that will only be contemptible if it remains unfinished as an act. "Acts must be pursued to their end. Whatever their starting point, the end will be beautiful. It is because it is not finished that an action is infamous" (Genet). The time of the song, the time of the writing of the act, enables a dimensioning, an a posteriori and the possibility of making a legend.

iii.

I decided to enter through the front door of what I will call, *Sartre's operation*, motivated by the best of intentions, which, by the way, we know what they lead to! *Saint Genet, comedian and martyr*, written in 1952 (curiously, the same year that *Frantz Fanon's Peau noire, masques blancs* was published by Gallimard), is a "literally monstrous work" says Eduardo Gruner, the prologue of the Argentine edition of *La Sartre*; he himself seems unaware of how much truth there is in this statement.

I quote:

> This is not simply because of its length (nearly seven hundred tight pages). Nor is it the fact that, originally intended as a prologue to the complete works of *Jean Genet, it* ended up almost exceeding the total number of pages of the complete works. With the effect that they are unthinkable today without the *supplementary reading* provided by this book.
>
> And concludes in a "violent innocence": "just as we cannot read Sophocles' *Oedipus Rex* today without thinking of Freud, we cannot read Genet without invoking Sartre".

Hopefully he is not right and we can still read Genet and Sophocles, at least partially, in the loopholes of these hermeneutics. Gruner concludes by equating this excess with a kind of *uneconomic and excessive potlatch* and likens it to *the inner experience* of Georges Bataille.

Over the years, I have learned to weigh things – and that includes theoretical productions – more by the effects they produce than by their supposed motives. Perhaps that is why I will allow myself not to overlook the subjective ravages of this "loving" operation. Although perhaps Sartre would be exempted by the narrator or narrators that Genet puts to play in his works, insofar as it is a betrayal of the beloved. But this would require a break with the bourgeois morality of homage.

Some attribute to this gesture of Sartre's that he saved Genet from life imprisonment; in the light of its effects, it is time to plan the benefits of this salvation. Sartre declares Genet dead: "And Genet is only a dead man; if he still seems to live, it is with that larval existence that certain peoples lend to their dead in the tombs . . . his death as an event of the past" (1967). The philosopher frames this death in what he calls "liturgical drama":

> "a child dies of shame and a rascal arises in his place", as a result of having been caught stealing at the age of ten. Thus he annuls all distinction between Genet and his characters, between author and narrator-protagonist.

I quote:

> She lives in terror of a repeat of the original crisis: she fears it like an epileptic seizure. Querelle could not get used to the never-formulated idea of being a monster. He considered, contemplated his past with a wry smile, frightened and affectionate at the same time, insofar as that past was mistaken for his own.

In April 1964, *Playboy* magazine interviewed Genet: "Did the extraordinary literary psychoanalysis that Sartre gave you upset you", the journalist asked:

> I was very upset because I saw myself undressed by someone else. I undress myself in my books, but at the same time I disguise myself with words, attitudes, certain choices, by means of a certain magic. I manage not to damage myself too much. But Sartre undressed me unceremoniously. My first impulse was to put the book down . . . it took me a while to get back to reading it.
>
> I felt unable to continue writing . . . Sartre's book created a vacuum that caused me to deteriorate psychologically . . . I remained in this unpleasant state for six years.

David Halperin (2000), who does not hesitate to describe Sartre's book as "impossibly tedious", (as does Susan Sontag) places the question in the dimension of power and authority: "In every biography, of course, the biographer certainly establishes a struggle with the biographer for the interpretative sovereignty of his life". Who has more authority to discover and specify the meaning of a life, the person who lived it or the person who writes it down? Erotics of domination, we ask.

And if, as Halperin says, "Foucault would have preferred the fictional re-tellings of him by Hervé Guibert – lurid as they are – to any biographical representation", alluding to David Macey's book *The Lives of Michel Foucault*, he would have been happier than if Sartre had essayed a fictionalisation of Genet. Although in the opinion of Marguerite Duras (1993), Sartre did not really "write". Not everyone who writes *writes*, but that is another matter. Some of Sartre's statements are striking because they are supposedly assertive, conclusive, "knowing". Sartre, like Lacan's sister Manene, knows:

> Genet is jealous of the singularity of the other and of his own singularity in the heart of the other. . . . Rather than let himself be redeemed by another, Genet

> will lose himself by his own means, he alone will achieve his singularity. [O] is nothing but the empty form of the singular in the face of the universal.

It is worth noting that Genet does not contest the truth of Sartre's assertions but that they are put forward by someone other than himself and the "naked" form, devoid of all art, of all ceremony, in the way he handles suffering. He will also reproach Sartre and Cocteau for having turned him into *a statue*.

iv.

Leo Bersani, in Chapter 4, "The Outlawed Gay", of the aforementioned book, refers to Gide and praises *The Immoralist* as a work at the antipodes of any psychology of desire, in the path of what he calls a *non-relational pederasty*, a theme he will take up again in *Sociability and Flirting*. The renunciation of "narcissistic autonomy", the possibility of a "pederasty without self", etc., would be questions to be dealt with, but this will not be the occasion. Bersani says that betrayal as an ethical necessity, "difficult and repugnant truth", is the obstacle to our interest in Jean Genet. And he goes further in terms of the writer's aims. According to Bersani, he would set out to "imagine a form of rebellion that has no relation whatsoever to the laws, categories, and values that it contests, and ideally, destroys". And he says:

> Let us try a more difficult position: Genet's use of the dominant terms of his culture (especially its ethical and sexual categories) does not seek to rework or subvert them, but to exploit their potential to erase cultural relationality itself.

Something of the social bond is strongly contested in this eroticism-turned-writing. However, we do not go along with a supposedly Freudian Bersani who reduces betrayal in Genet to its mythical, oedipal dimension, in which a third party "saves" the subject from the "copulatory fullness"; we do not see it in the same way. Nor when he makes of the fantasy of the narrador in *Pompas fúnebres* to enter the anus of the dead loved one, a reversal, an inversion of the return to the maternal womb proposed by Sandor Ferenczi.

George Bataille, for his part, condemns the absence of "ultimate loyalty" in Genet's work, and the term he uses to speak of its absence is curious: "sovereignty". Genet's work renounces all sovereignty, whereas Bataille's sovereignty is given in communication. Genet does not communicate; he isolates himself in a false sovereignty, in mistrust. Once again, although in a different way, Genet seems to be used to exemplify a theory, in this case to contrast it, moreover, with that of another philosopher (Sartre).

Didier Eribon (2004) claims not to seek "to restore the real Genet but to extract from some of his texts an ethics of minority subjectification". One of the merits, and only one, of Eribon's text is that it is the rescue of the notion of *shame* in Genet's writing. And although with many qualms "one swallow does not make a summer", he borrows from Lacan the neologism *hontologie*, which the publisher translates very badly as *vergonzology*; losing the interplay between shame and logos. Shame that appears when "the social gaze taxonomically qualifies the individual and pins him on the panel of infamous species". This is an obvious nod to Foucault's *The Lives of Infamous Men*. We thus enter, in Genet's words, the "universe of the irremediable. It is the same as the one we are in, but with one particularity: instead of acting and knowing ourselves to be acting, we know ourselves to be acted upon".

We have already shown in *Of a power that is not exercised*[5] how Jean Allouch (2005) writes in *Avergonzados*, recalling the first meetings of psychoanalysts and trans people, from their shame, when:

> "Jacques-Marie Lacan, who received a transsexual for his presentation of the sick, had words that I would not wish to reproduce, shame on myself for having so late taken the position I am stating here, shame on the Freudian movement . . .". And he adds: Everything happened as if Jacques-Marie Lacan had forgotten his ternary, and thanks to this forgetfulness, the old "reality" came out of his pocket. "Reality", the same one that his ternary was refusing. And things took their course. Lacan's forgetfulness, or the effects of a dominant discourse that constitutes us and causes "the unwary to err" in this way too?

Manuel Hernández (2013), in "La rotura o la vergüenza", analyses the shame of calling oneself a psychoanalyst and the shame of calling oneself a Mexican. He rescues the ontological status that Lacan gives to shame, "Ontic problematic that goes through a critical problem of the register of nomination. Of inscription as a subjectivising operation".

It takes up Gayatri Chakravorty Spivac's approach to "epistemic violence", which she understands as the alteration, negation, and in extreme cases – such as that of colonisations – the extinction of the meanings of the everyday, juridicial, and symbolic life of individuals and groups. "The consequence is silence", says Spivac. Genet bore witness to this in the six years that followed the appearance of Sartre's "Saint Genet . . .". As a non-anecdotal fact, it is worth remembering that *Diary of the Dragon* had been dedicated *to Sartre*. I would call this episode: *Of the non-equivalence of tributes*.

Manuel Hernández makes a certain "rescue" of shame from the side of the analysand confronted with the discourse of the master:

> Doing an analysis confronts everyone with their own shame. The shame generated by the object a in the place of production arises from the discourse of the master, but from that same hole, Lacan says, the master signifier can in turn arise again, as happens in the discourse of the analyst. Let us clarify something, the discourse of the analyst does not write the end of analysis, the production of the master signifier S_1 is in no way conclusive of a psychoanalysis, but an ongoing operation.

At the end of his work, Hernández asks himself: "can there be a free sacrifice of a piece of the self, without any kind of inscription"?

What kind of nomination, what kind of inscription was left for Jean Genet after Sartre's essay, that of a saint, is that a possible inscription, did it suit Genet? He will say something about the name when he discovers the widespread nature of the theft, its non-uniqueness. Poetry rescues it: "Poetry resides in its heightened awareness of its quality as a thief. *It may be that the awareness of any other quality capable of becoming essential to the point of giving you a name is equally poetry*". Or in another passage:

> now that I reread myself I have forgotten those boys, there is nothing left of them but this attribute which I have sung. (. . . I have not sought excuses or justification for them. I wanted them to have the right to the honours of the Name.

Threads are woven that perhaps allow us, by means of detours, approximations, and distancing, to generate other possibilities of thought around the questions that summon me. Contrary to many texts and papers in which the text or texts that move the discourse are placed at the beginning to facilitate the application of theory – even psychoanalytic theory – I intend to give Genet the floor, finally, so that he may show with his words the inadequacies of any reading, of any commentary.

If it is true that Genet makes waste the object of desire, it is also true that there will be an unassimilable, indomitable remainder to be respected, to be left to be.

V.

> "I call violence a resting audacity in love with dangers".
>
> —Jean Genet

I would like to read *Diary of the Thief* as one reads *Fragments of a Discourse on Love* by Roland Barthes (saving the differences, which are many, by the way), in "packets of sentences".

From the *Diary* . . .

> My victory is verbal and I owe it to the sumptuousness of the terms, but blessed be the misery that advises me to make such choices.
>
> It seemed to me that men, the hard men, were a kind of feminine mist in which I would like to be lost in order to feel even more like a solid block.
>
> In this diary I do not wish to disguise the other reasons that made me a thief, the simplest being the need to eat; but my choice was never influenced by rebellion, bitterness, anger, or any other such feeling. With a maniacal care, a jealous care, I prepared my adventure as one prepares a bed, a room for love: the creature has imprisoned me.

Regarding poetic emotion:

> It left in my soul a kind of wake of restlessness that was gradually fading. . . . I remained attentive to capture those wandering moments that seemed to me to be searching, as a soul in pain searches for a body, for a conscience to capture and feel them. When they have found it, they cease. The poet exhausts the world. But if he produces another, it can only be the fruit of his own reflection.

Of *Diary of the Thief*, he will say that it is "the pursuit of the Imposible Nullity". Of *eroticism:*

> Each of my lovers gives rise to a crime novel. They are therefore the elaboration of an erotic ceremonial, of a sometimes very long mating, these nocturnal and dangerous adventures in which I let myself be dragged along by shady heroes.

The writer remembers Guy, one of his lovers, as "a passionate temperament, a fiery life" . . . as someone who "knows how to ruin himself in one night for himself or for a friend". From *Funeral Pomps*:

> When she teams up with a young Hitlerite and an executioner, enemies of her dead young lover, to give an account of their love through betrayal:
>
> We seemed to be alone, characters with no past and no future . . . united to each other not by a succession of events but by the play of a gracious gratuitousness, the gratuitousness of the poetic fact. We were there in the fog of the world.
> Of *writing:*
>
> I didn't see clearly the reasons for my choice, the meaning of which perhaps appears to me today because I have to write it down. I think I needed to delve deeper, to pierce a mass of language in which my thoughts would be at ease. Perhaps I wanted to accuse myself in my own language. . . . To be a thief in my own country, to become one and to justify myself for being one by using the language of the stolen – which is me in person because of the importance of language – was to give this quality of thief the opportunity to become unique. It made me a foreigner.
>
> To conclude:
>
> Finally, the greater, the more complete, the more completely my guilt is in your eyes, the greater will be my freedom. . . . Thanks to my guilt I gained the right to intelligence. Too many people who have no right to that, he thinks. They have not paid for that right with such an undertaking that thinking becomes indispensable for your salvation.
>
> Perhaps it is time to do, to be silent.

Notes

1 *Billy Bud, Sailor* (1924) is an unfinished work by Herman Melville (2013). The novel tells the story of a sailor who is recruited from a ship called "Human Rights" – names in Melville have their importance. This sailor is, first of all, of a very particular beauty, and he assumes a very particular subjective position. We know almost nothing of his own history; he is a character who has no history, but his position on the ship generates very unique relationships, which have little to do with what is traditionally shown about relationships on merchant ships of that time or of this time. He finds himself in opposition to Claggart, the ship's master-at-arms, a tyrannical being, who represents a completely arbitrary use of power. As is to be expected, Billy Budd generates a very particular eroticism in his shipmates, which makes him the object of love and hate at the same time. Of course it ends badly, he dies by hanging, accused of a treason he did not commit.

2 Several authors have pointed out the subjective inconvenience of the dilution of erotics into a single category or nomination, except for political purposes (more than justified, by the way).

3 Love that will be problematised in other works as essentially heterosexual, because of its historicisation in the framework of what Louis-George Tin (2012) called *The Invention of Heterosexual Culture*.

4 However, I cannot and do not wish to overlook Eve Kosofsky Sedgwick's (1998) insightful point in *Epistemology of the Closet* about the ambiguity of this destabilising potential and its counterpart of masculinist reinforcement as a possible derivative of homoeroticism: "Is desire for other men the preserver of masculinist hierarchies in Western culture or, on the contrary, one of its greatest threats?

5 Of a power that is not exercised, p. 36.

Chapter 5

Of saying as practice

> a rough and sweet liquor works in the throats that sing of the disaffection of the intelligence
> the astuteness of some knowledge that ignores the derisory of itself
>
> —Fernando Barrios, *desnacidos* (unpublished)

Saying psychoanalysis: The effects of writing

The author of the following paper – which was intended as a paper for a future colloquium – chooses not to use bibliographical references or punctuation marks in the conventional sense.

Warning

the text will make room for a number of commonplaces of psychoanalysis that have become commonplace, even banal things that have become banal, repeated everyday commonplaces, in the hope that perhaps bringing them up again – in a palimpsest of un(re)quoted quotations – will give us back something of that first radicality in this practice of writing I won't quote almost anyone, much less anyone or a few of them, much less textual and with bibliographical reference, I will not quote almost anyone, or only a few at any rate – and when I do, most of the time I won't make it known, I will appropriate their saying, which is the same as saying: I will submit myself to it – so that it flows . . . to say psychoanalysis and in appropriating myself I will confuse myself with that other of the saying that writes to me My design would be that it should be a monstrox text, a Frankenstein text, made of remains in a proliferating progression of jouissance, a failed and pretentious in-human pastiche, a sewer text of things said and heard, written by half-saying, made of anachronisms and false contestations with only one certainty: its rhetorical impossibility: its rhetorical impossibility . . . this will be the only stop one of a working progress because there is nothing more eccentric of me than myself surrounded by a deci-writing that makes any authorship impossible although some of this eccentricity finds its limit in the saying, since it has been said that the unconscious is articulated by what comes from being to the saying . . . of course a being

DOI: 10.4324/9781003710295-5

in lack of being in lack then to confirm that in psychoanalysis when one says I will not do such a thing it is an announcement that it will be done: let us begin with a quotation:

> if the poem makes the saying less silly . . . as Lacan suggests in the epilogue to the edition of *The Four Concepts* . . . let us try something of that saying without pretending that the poetry marching in step with the question it is trying to produce produces – eventually – the question is said in Lituraterre . . . or we will make it be said because that is what we believe it is about, a saying and a practice, a saying of that practice which is the sayingwriting we echo the fact that there is a saying that moves us writing is not the same as saying we know it and even contrary to what intuition would have us believe the writing precedes the saying . . . logically of course . . . effects of language

Writing plays its part in the saying informs the saying, says Jean Allouch, a reader of Lacan. A writing gives form to this saying that we decided by writing

To say as the continuation of a writing by other means?

I write a piece of writing that writes me when I write it, I am that piece of writing that is me" I wrote some time ago because "without saying there are not many things, almost none" said someone somewhere, but that does not mean that this writing will stop hiding in my saying, offering itself in the truest way because although there is nothing more than writing in the half-saying of that writing, it is far from being useless because it is also a practice of charlatanism, because "there is nothing more than phrases . . . what does not prevent (. . . from having consequences", that saying something is about the impossible to say because "saying is something else to talk about which does not prevent them . . . from having consequences" to say something is about the impossible to say because "saying is something other than speaking" To say the impossible, that is writing. To read what to say writes is a game and is also freedom, it is "to open up an abyss to thought".

We know of Jacques Lacan's enormous resistance to writing, to the passage from his own writing to another kind of writing that would take up this saying, and we also know of the not always happy – and often unhappy – vicissitudes in the passage-establishment of his seminars.

Establishing the saying, is this a desirable policy?

There is a politics in writing that always biases the saying towards one side or the other, that places emphasis and executes omissions and distortions, that fixes – what was not intended – in a conceptual mode that coheres, that editorialises, that textualises, that establishes – perhaps this is one of the reasons why Lacan could not have accompanied Derrida in his "there is nothing outside the text" It is not about that writing in psychoanalysis, the text is already a political operation, a political operation of writing some time ago I read from a literary critic something that made me review what operations I was subjecting my poetic or allegedly poetic practice to, he said: there are no books of poetry, there is a book operation by which poetry is grouped together in a false unity – all unity is only imaginary, perhaps something of that order also happens in psychoanalysis, but writing will be something else in psychoanalysis, it will be "the letter that kills without any intervention of the spirit" . . . we call it the unconscious, there is a practice of saying that Freud inaugurates, which is not the same as saying that he creates or invents it, or perhaps it is, if we extend the notion of creation or invention to taking something from one field to another to those small and not at all minor displacements by which something from one supposed field is taken to another, not without consequences, something of this mode of saying already inhabited poetry and worldly saying, a mode of saying that Freud radicalises, perhaps knowingly or not, pointing to its (im)posibility:

To say everything that comes into one's head or spirit without leaving anything out . . . it is known to be (im)possible . . . hence its necessity this impossibility says of a real that can only be barely said but which we will not be able to get rid of if we do not want to make a theory of psychoanalysis psychoanalysis as theory that is what theory seeks for Lacan "to get rid of" to get rid of not having anything to do with any jouissance with any real in the saying . . . there is a point of theoretical impossibility of psychoanalysis to locate the saying in the writing to establish it to stabilise it: writing in this way is a kind of secondary elaboration like that to which dreams are subjected once the writing has been re-established.

the end of bookish culture, already announced by Ivan Illich and Steiner and so many others, generates panics that are also epistemic and political "cultural" panics, i.e.: class Eurocentric i.e., colonial i.e., white class-merited and a long etcetera alphabetism will say Allouch panic that ignores unlettered or otherwise literate cultures in another relation to language where the oral or writing is not alphabetic of a saying writes-inscribes that saying sayings that make that rewrite each time saying magical sayings of real power effectively respected and feared.

"Bookish reading can now be clearly recognised as the phenomenon of an epoch and not as a logically necessary step in the progress towards the rational use of the alphabet; as one mode, among several" says Illich in *The vineyard* of the text and that setting in variety: one among several, seems to me an operation to be done with all the pretended universals, to make diverse or pluriverse or multiverse what is pretended to be universal as a first step towards opening other possibilities other Something of a deontologisation of the world – another universal to drop from an antimetaphysics of this invention called the West where the sun never stops falling West that makes etymological family with decadent and with corpse

"Omnium expetendorum prima est sapientia. Of all things to be sought, the first is wisdom". This is how Jerome Taylor translates the main sentence of the Didascalicon of Hugo of St. Victor, written around 1128" says Ivan Illich right at the beginning of his text and then already there he places us in front of a very first issue: the relation to knowledge; relation to and the very notion of knowledge that in psychoanalysis does not cease to be a problem, does not cease not to be resolved in its relation to the truth, but not only . . . unconscious knowledge that inhabits the language, that produces it which is the language, the language in its materiality, producer of bodies that are re-written in relation to knowledge that will give rise to discourses that are social ties that by a quarter turn turn other agents relocating other production and truth at the same time as signifier, master knowledge, subject and object.

In this way, the question will be: to which discourse does a discourse respond, corresponds to a discourse? say as a speech effect . . . halfway, between writing and speaking Saying psychoanalysis will not be identical to analytic discourse unless we renounce saying outside the analytic device Something of that discourse can permeate saying outside the analytic act and its device on condition of other renunciations and warnings renunciation of university discourse in the first place what is easier to say than to do renunciation of making knowledge master and which could imply abandoning oneself as much as one can to a saying that is said by saying oneself – and also by saying without catechist pretensions – conceptual precisions and formal and formalist rigours ranging from the relation of quotation to the argument of authority – magister dixit – which we could play at calling it master of knowledge and which could imply an abandoning oneself as much as one can to a saying that is said by saying oneself – and also by saying without catechist pretensions. The argument of authority – magister dixit – which we could play with by calling it master dixit argumentative order, etc., etc. . . . but all that is not enough either . . .

are we ready to tolerate this immixion of another decirescribing in our spaces of writing? to say that it will never be direct we know it by saying that "it rescinds its subject" says Lacan, it leaves it without effect, it makes it the effect of that saying. Saying that comes from what is saidwritten.

The "ex-iste to what is said" occupies an eccentric place with respect to what is said. said that will remain forgotten behind what is said in what is heard in what is heard in what is written that will blur the frontiers, the borders between writing and visuality, between virtuality and presence, between materialities of different orders, between authorship and the collective agency of enunciation, between subjective fragments and work . . . more on the side of pharmakon than of remedium, a saying that cures and poisons, alleviates and pursues, allowing neither stabilisation nor any kind of health. To say pharmakon is to say that it is neither divine verb nor self-knowledge but asceticism of the spirit, which is also body . . . exercise of the self . . . de-conoce. "Disknow thyself" I wrote some time ago in a booklet I called "desaforismos, apócrifos y otras herjías" (Disaphorisms, apocryphalisms and other heresies).

a saying perhaps closer to the poetic than to the essay or the narrative, a "speculative fabulation" as Donna Haraway would have it? And it will not be about expecting *illuminations of the self* as Hugo St. Victor, read by Ivan Illich, would want: "The effort of study that Hugo teaches is a commitment to an activity through which the reader's own "I" will light up and shine" but rather, in any case, an *illumination* that, as Jean Allouch points out, differs from interpretation without losing its relation to it by substituting itself in that: "the image says and language figures" imagines by imagining the real and realising the imaginary illumination as a rupture as an abrupt access to a knowledge other by a succession of illuminations or by occasions in which the image burns in the encounter with the real, as George Didi-Hubermann puts it, because following the chamines of the letter we burn "in a fire that is lit everywhere". Perhaps not so far from the inspired and illuminated sayings and writings of madmen and madwomen, why not? Perhaps it is expecting too much, perhaps it is expecting the impossible . . . but if it is psychoanalysis, what else could be expected?

Psychoanalysis and literature: Genealogy of an unresolved tension

The relationship between literature and psychoanalysis does not go without saying. That is to say: it is not evident, although it may seem so. There is *an unresolved tension* every time we try to operate in the crossings between their fields. Here are just a few notes.

The equivocation of a Freud awarded the Goethe Prize for Literature speaks of an overlapping to be cleared up and at the same time not to stop (un)doing. If we do not give in to the application of psychoanalysis, to its temptation, something becomes tense and opens up possible drifts that concern both the epistemic and the methodological, both dimensions of a *politics of saying* in psychoanalysis.

If we take over Jacques Lacan's felicitous expression in *L'etourdit (*1972): *psychoanalysis as a practice of saying*, if we take up this post, we must try to account for the fact that there is a writing that logically causes the saying which in turn – eventually – can become writing.

It is then that writing, saying, signifier, letter, semblance and jouissance, enunciation, discourse, are put to play a game of multiple, non-dialectical relays, in signifying progression-digression towards a real hole that makes impossible any pretension of dominion over that which speaks to us.

Literature then becomes litura-terra, crossing out and lifting up, trace and trace between jouissance and knowledge . . . littoral and remainder.

If, as Jean Michel Rabaté points out: "literature inhabits theory from the beginning, and makes it tremble, waver with respect to its own status", then the very notion of fields and crossings becomes denser and involves the literary in the very constitution of the knowledge of psychoanalysis. It then becomes necessary to produce some kind of genealogy of this *productive density*.

Only if we look at Freud's readings, a very extensive list of authors makes his effects evident: Sophocles, Virgil, Shakespeare, Swift, Milton, Spencer, George Eliot, Kipling, Kingsley, Haggard, Max Müller, Charles Dickens, Balzac, Flaubert, Zola, Maupassant, Rabelais, Molière, Voltaire, Rousseau, Victor Hugo, Pascal, Alexandre Dumas junior, Dostoevsky, Tolstoy and Merejkovsky, Ibsen, Kleist, Uhland, Grabbe, the Brothers Grimm, Goethe, anonymous legends *[Nibelungenlied]*, Bürger, Christian Fürchtegott Gellert, Herder, Kortum, Lessing, Lichtenberg. So also Fritz Reuter, Heinrich von Kleist, Grillparzer, Theodor Herlz, Gottfried Keller, Joseph Viktor von Scheffel, and Arthur Schnitzler, among others (Motta, 2013). Lacan's list would probably be even longer (Estrín, 2002), and to that we would have to add the multiple readings whose effects are not recorded, although they do their work.

Since Freud, some kind of narrativity not only inhabits, but enables the very emergence of psychoanalysis. Mythical narrativity of Oedipus, anthropological of the primitive horde, biological of sexual difference or philosophical in the very notion of the unconscious. Narratives that will fall or give way to another discourse, not without these underpinnings. Not only is this narrativity not outside a clinic, but it constitutes it not only without piercing itself, not only without failing each time. There is a rhetorical impossibility that hacks all pretensions of univocity of meaning, when saying becomes letter.

In Lacan, despite the fact that he does not consider himself to be sufficiently-

In a poetic mind, something moves towards a saying that is closer to the poetic and the aphoristic. Jacques Lacan's rhetoric itself tries not to tear apart the writing that causes it, as well as that which it produces.

In 1965 he says of his seminar:

> . . . it unfolds from the parenthesis, the suspense and then from its often very uncomfortable resumption, you should recognise in it, once again, the structure of writing.
>
> (Jacques Lacan, 1986)

The very notion of subject is in question, if we take into account his statement in the preface to the English edition of *The Four Concepts of Psychoanalysis* (Lacan, 1965–1966): "A certificate says that I was born. I repudiate this certificate: I am not a poet, but a poem. A poem that is being written, even though it has the air of being a subject".

As beings of writing with no other ontological consistency, we are spoken and enjoyed by a language that is spoken in each person, it remains to be seen in what way. Thus, if we were to revisit from psychoanalysis – without pretending to find there what we already know – some of: Edgar Allan Poe, Dickens, Dostoevsky, Shakespeare, Gide, Joyce, Beckett, and Sade. Lewis Carroll and Marguerite Duras among others. Like Lacan's work with François Cheng on Chinese poetry and thought over the years, we could at least follow the trail of this work – not "with the literary" but *of the literary* in psychoanalysis, *between criticism and the clinic.*

Not so long ago, I discovered a text that says something of what I am proposing, regarding the problematisation of the psychoanalysis/literature relation: Pierre Bayard (2009), *Can literature be applied to psychoanalysis?* With a provocative title, Bayard inverts the terms and power relations in the operation of the application of one field to another. This is how I read its title, in the face of the author's warning about the *impossibility* of the wager as early as Fernando Pessoa's passage in *The Book of Disquiet:* "All problems are insoluble. Essentially, the existence of a problem presupposes the non-existence of a solution".

Even Bayard will say it directly:

> The purpose of this book is to try to understand the reasons why the method of reading that I invented and patiently perfected over the years – a method that

> consists in applying literature to psychoanalysis – turned out, against all expectations, to be a failure.

This perhaps also tells us that there are power relations between one field and another, epistemic primacies, discursive hegemonies, etc., which does not prevent us from trying out other ways of conceiving the relationship between fields.

And from the reading of Homer's *Iliad*:

> What these opening pages of Homer show, or at any rate confirm, is that writers have not waited for the advent of the modern age to take an interest in the psychological conflicts and bonds of desire that interweave between beings. Like the other heroes of the Trojan War, for whom analogous trances could easily be found, Achilles and Agamemnon are not monolithic characters. On the contrary, they are torn between complex feelings, some of which are directly described, and some of which are suggested and assumed by the actions that result from them and the interactions in which they are embedded. And although the writer does not subject them to a psychological analysis as such, he does stage them with sufficient precision for some singular reflection to emerge or be inspired by them.

And then he warns us about the application of psychoanalysis to literature:

> Well, applied literature has been created precisely against this kind of procedure, whether one is looking for an unconscious significance in the literary work or trying to show how the author has anticipated modern psychological theories. The author's attempt to show how the author has anticipated modern psychological theories. For in either case, it is through an external theory, and not produced from the work, that the work is read, and this oriented reading prevents him from developing his own theory.
>
> The fact of perceiving the work through an established system, whatever the interest of this system may be, has the consequence of not giving importance to what it can bring of originality to the reflection on the psyche, and therefore not giving it all the attention it deserves.
>
> Indeed, when Homer presents the feelings of the two characters, he speaks neither of conflict nor of inconscious, but, for example, of a hero who "argues between two things" or who "turns his thoughts over in his mind" before a goddess comes to reconcile him with himself. In the poet, therefore, there is a personal attempt to produce a representation of our psychological functioning, an attempt which should be respected and studied as such.
>
> In fact, there are two ways of not neglecting the representations that the literature of antiquity, but also that of later centuries, offer us of psychic reality. The first, which we will try to avoid, consists, not without a certain feeling of superiority, in taking an interest in the writers' proposals, perceived as successively surpassed stages, in order to elaborate psychic models. This is against the

> background of a progressive conception of the history of ideas, which would gradually approach, with varying degrees of approximation, an ultimate truth.

And precise:

> The second way, that of applied literature, consists in taking these models seriously, not forcibly placing them in a progression and accepting the idea that they are not necessarily inferior in precision or poetic beauty to those that the theorists of the psyche will later elaborate. That the great reading systems of the nineteenth and twentieth centuries, of which psychoanalysis is a part, are not necessarily inferior in precision or poetic beauty to those that theorists of the psyche will later elaborate.
>
> The most representative, they have not been killed or killed off, but they are still alive and deserve to be given interest, in their own right and not as mere stages.

There is one point that seems to us of particular interest since it intersects with Lacan's conception of theory in psychoanalysis. In *From an Other to the Other*, he says: "We have a relation to theory to the extent that it is lightened by the introduction of the function of the plus-de-jouir" (2008). We read this initially ambiguous statement as meaning that theory seeks to disengage itself from its relation to jouissance, to have nothing to do with it. This is why in psychoanalysis either it is not theory or it is a very particular kind of theory.

Since Freud ([1906] 1989a) and his analysis of W. Jensen's *Gradiva*, we know that literature allows other ways of doing with jouissance, it is a particular *erotic operation*:

> The poet does not let us trace the influences that made our hero fall into that state of estrangement respecting the woman; he only puts us on the track that this behaviour is not explained by his (constitutional) disposition, but rather encloses within itself a piece of fantastic subjective necessity – we would complete on our own: erotic.

> An erotic operation that is also a doing with madness:

> Miss Zoé herself seems to share our conception of the young archaeologist's delirium, for the complacency she expresses at the end of her "ruthless, prolix and sobering sermon" can hardly have any other foundation than her proclivity to refer his interest in Gradiva to her own person from the very beginning. It was what she would never have expected of him and yet discerned as such despite all the disguises of delirium. In him, on the other hand, the psychic treatment she had given him had its beneficial effect; he felt liberated, for now the delirium was replaced by that of which it could only be a disfigured and inadequate reflection.

And in relation to psychoanalysis as a *system of reading* to which Bayard alludes, there are those who raise the crux of the matter. Thus, Nicolás Garayalde (2018) says in *Literature and psychoanalysis: towards a theory of reading:* "the contribution that psychoanalysis can make to the field of literary studies is neither in criticism nor in literature but in the theory and epistemology of reading".

But in order not to do what Bayard warns us against, let us go to what he says:

> This book is less devoted to the presentation of a new method than to the difficulty of theorising or, if you like, to the secrets of manufacture that writing, in its security, tends to conceal. Every critical text is based on a series of reductions of the work and approximations to thought which are necessary for its existence, but which cost literature dearly. So the precise study of what goes wrong in a particular method can contribute, like certain silences of the analyst in the cure, to restoring to the works a little of their *freedom of speech.*
>
> (Italics are mine)

Bayard goes so far as to say that what psychoanalysis does to literature is a poisoned gift:

> Thus, behind the mask of praise, the theory of endopsychic knowledge is a poisoned gift that psychoanalysis gives to literature. For praise is murderous. Under the façade of a tribute to the intuition of writers, what is subtly established is a considerable limitation of their capacity for invention. It is true that they are recognised as having a knowledge, superior in addition – at least in terms of its anteriority to that of science – but this is immediately limited, channelled, framed. What literature knows is the psychoanalysis to come.

Later he will say:

> What radically separates the applied literature from other critical methodologies inspired by psychoanalysis is thus the question that is asked of the work. . . . The question is what this work can bring new to our reflection on the psyche and, therefore, what original thought it is the repository of.

And then it will be a question of

> the question posed to literature by applied literature is no longer on the side of the unconscious meaning of the work but on the side of its knowledge, or better still – for this is a dynamism to be translated – of its virtual thought.

Personally, I prefer the first formulation: the question points to the *knowledge of the work*. The notion of thought in psychoanalysis – at least since Lacan's considerations in this regard – remains problematic or to be problematised. Knowledge of the work that is not equivalent to knowledge of its author, by the way. Remember

Lacan's comment to Marguerite Duras: "Marguerite Duras turns out to know without me what I teach". And he bases his homage: "that the practice of the letter converges with the use of the unconscious, is what I will testify to by paying homage to her" (Lacan, 2001).

There is in the practice of handwriting a knowledge which, not knowing itself, works. Let us return to Bayard, who, tightening the threads even further, proposes:

> this thought is irreducible to the unconscious sense constructed by the Freudian model, which does not exhaust its propositions. It consists of a specific capacity to read the psychic world, capable of sculpting it in an original way. And that, in this sense, it deserves to be studied in its own right.

Despite being highly critical of Freud and Lacan, Bayard knows in the latter "the way in which he constantly invents concepts from his reading of works, clearly links him to what we call applied literature". Paraphrasing Jean Allouch (2015) in his text "To speak is already to write", we would say: *To read is already to write* . . . Lacan the reader, gives a full account of this.

In relation to poetry, Lacan refers to it on many occasions, in tension with the practice of analysis. In the seminar *Psychosis*, he will say:

> There is poetry every time a writing introduces us to a world different from our own, and . . . makes it ours as well. . . . Poetry is the creation of a subject who assumes a new order of symbolic relation with the world.
>
> (Lacan, 1984c)

In *The Four Concepts*, Lacan refers to the condensed dimension of the poem:

> "More hidden than you think," he says, "for it is not enough for me to bring forth the scythe that Jupiter uses to flood the earth with the blood of Cronus."
>
> (Lacan, 1986)

In *L'insu*, Lacan (1977) will point out that: "poetry (. . .) is the effect of meaning, but also the effect of the hole". In "Variants of the cure-type" (1985):

> There is only poetry, I have told you, which allows for interpretation. That is why I do not go further, in my technique, than what she claims. I am not poâte enough.
>
> Or in "Lituraterre" (1971):
>
> Between centre and absence, between knowledge and jouissance, there is a coastline that only turns to the literal if they can make this same turn at all times. It is only in this way that they can be taken by the agent that sustains it. . . . What is revealed by my vision of the alluvium in terms of what dominates the

crossing out, is that when it is produced among the clouds, it is conjugated with its source. It is precisely to the clouds that Aristophanes calls me to discover what happens to the signifier, that is to say, the semblant par excellence, if it is through their rupture that this effect rains down from them, when what was there matter in suspension is precipitated.

In "Television" (1977):

The virtue that I designate with the gaya ciencia is an example of it, to show what it consists in: not in understanding, in biting into meaning, but in passing as close to it as possible.

And to take Heidegger's (1987) warning in *On the Way to Speech:* "For now I see the danger even more clearly: the language of our conversation continually destroys the possibility of deciring that of which we speak," we wonder whether something similar will not happen with the language with which we say-write psychoanalysis.

François Cheng (2000), who had years of meetings with Lacan, tells us that the latter was extremely curious about Chinese writing:

What fascinates Lacan, however, are these written signs as a system. *A system that is at the service of the word, while keeping a distance from it.* As each ideogram forms an autonomous and invariable unit, its signifying power is only slightly diluted in the chain. Thus, being capable of faithfully transcribing the word, the system can also, by a whole process of voluntary ellipsis and free combination, engender within itself an open play, especially in poetic language where, within a sign and between signs, the central Void plays at pulverising the domain of one-dimensional linearity.

(Emphasis added)

And he concludes:

In this connection, let us remember that I left Lacan around 1974 to devote myself precisely to the writing of a work on Chinese poetic writing. This work, published in 1977, attracted Lacan's full attention. In a letter dated 22 April 1977, he wrote to me 1977, he writes to me: "I took your book into account in my last seminar, saying that interpretation – that is to say, what the analyst must do – must be poetic".

Something of how to do otherwise with emptiness, perhaps we can also learn from poetic speech.

Bibliography

Ahmed, Sara (2006). *Queer phenomenology*. London: Duke University Press.

Ahmed, Sara (2015). *La política cultural de las emociones*. Mexico: UNAM, PUEG.

Ahmed, Sara (2018). "Queer fragility", in *Journal of Literary Theory and Comparative Literature and Comparative Literature* (18), pp. 196–208. Available at: https://www.raco.cat/index.php/452F/article/view/333760/424621

Ahmed, Sara (2019). *The promise of happiness. A cultural critique of the imperative of joy*. Buenos Aires: Caja Negra Editora.

Allouch, Jean (1996). "L'éthification de la psychanalyse", in *Calamité Cahiers de l'Unebévue*. Paris, EPEL.

Allouch, Jean (1998). *El psicoanálisis una erotología de pasaje*. Ed Literales.

Allouch, Jean (1999). "Welcoming gay and lesbian studies", in *Edelp: Litoral*, 27.

Allouch, Jean (2000). "Jacques Lacan analysing himself", in *Acheronta*, December. Available at: https://www.acheronta.org/acheronta12/lacan-en.htm

Allouch, Jean (2004). *The shadow of your dog. Psychoanalytic discourse. Lesbian discourse*. Buenos Aires: El cuenco de plata.

Allouch, Jean (2005). "Avergonzados", in *Imago Agenda*. Buenos Aires. Available at: http://www.imagoagenda.com/articulo.asp?idarticulo=440

Allouch, Jean (2007). *Is psychoanalysis a spiritual exercise? Response to Michel Foucault*. Buenos Aires: El cuenco de plata – Ediciones literales.

Allouch, Jean (2009). *The sex of the master. El erotismo desde Lacan*. Buenos Aires: El cuenco de plata.

Allouch, Jean (2013). *Prisoners of the great other. Divine interference i*. Buenos Aires: El cuenco de plata.

Allouch, Jean (2015). *Heterotica i. On the sexual non-relationship in the Ancients according to Foucault*. Montevideo: Seminar. 25 and 26 July.

Allouch, Jean (2017). *No heterosexual relationship*. Mexico: Epeele-Literales.

Allouch, Jean (2020). *Interview with Stéphane Breton*. Paris: 21 March. Translation from French by Itzel Casillas Avalos and Jaime Ruíz Noé.

Allouch, Jean et al. (2019). *Con piel de Lobo. Cien años de una neurosis infantil*. Montevideo: Escolios.

Andrés, Rodrigo (2006). *Herman Melville, power and love between men*. University of Valencia. Available at: https://www.ub.edu/adhuc/publicacions/herman-melville-poder-y-amor-entre-ho

Arboleda Ríos, Paola (2011). "Ser o estar 'queer' en Latinoamérica? El devenir emancipador", in Lemebel, Perlongher and Arenas Iconos (eds.). *Revista de Ciencias Sociales*, n. 39. Ecuador: Facultad Latinoamericana de Ciencias Sociales.

Assandri, José (2008). "La saga del fetichismo en La psicopatología revisitada", in *ñacate*, 1. Available at: http://www.revistanacate.com/revista/numero-1/

Assandri, José (2011). "Ser justos con Lacan?", in *Coloquio Raíces expuestas. Cuadernos Claroscuro. Lacan, reenchanting the work?* Costa Rica.

Ayouch, Thamy (2018). "From the binary to the multiple: Gendered subjectivations in Candomblé". Available at: https://www.cairn.info/revue-cliniques-mediterraneennes-2018-1-page-159.htm

Ayouch, Thamy (2020). *Psychoanalysis and hybridity. Gender, coloniality, subjectivations.* Mexico: Ed. Navarra.

Ayouch, Thamy (2021). "Conversations with e-dictions justine", 30 May. Available at: https://e-diccionesjustine-elp.net/interview-with-thamy-ayouch/

Balcarce, Gabriela (2016–2017). "Algunas reflexiones sobre la espectralidad en el pensamiento de Jacques Derrida", in *Convivium* 29/30. Buenos Aires: Universidad de Buenos Aires, pp. 203–216.

Barrios, Fernando (1993). "Ser y parecer. Identidad sexual y narcisismo en Narcisismo", in *Montevideo, Roca Viva*, pp. 49–60.

Barrios, Fernando (1995). "Felisberto Hernández, a journey from pain to creation. creation. Analysis of the short story La pelota", in *Revista Uruguaya de Psicoanálisis*, 82.

Barrios, Fernando (2005). *El sótano y otros cuentos.* Montevideo: Editorial Atlántida.

Barrios, Fernando (2015). *Textual vortex.* Box-book. Montevideo: Author's Edition.

Barrios, Fernando (2017a). "Campo queer, estado de situación", in *Revista Relaciones.* Vol. 399. Montevideo.

Barrios, Fernando (2017b). "Of a power that is not exercised", in *Presentation in two Malestares en la ciudad. Five nights of analysts in the polis.* Montevideo, Ediciones de la fuga and Witz editor, pp. 75–89.

Barrios, Fernando (2018a). "History of violence or violence of history?", in *Colloquium Racialized Eros*, 24 November. Montevideo: École lacanienne de psychanalyse. Available at: Montevideo. https://e-diccionesjustine-elp.net/eros-racialised/

Barrios, Fernando (2018b). "Saying of psychoanalysis. Writing effects". Available at: https://e-diccionesjustine-elp.net/practicas-del-decir/

Barrios, Fernando (2018c). "What heterosexuality owes to psychoanalysis". Available at: http://www.revistanacate.com/lo-que-la-heterosexualidad-le-debe-al-psicoanalisis/

Barrios, Fernando (2019). "Jean Genet, a practice of saying or a certain kind of magic". Available at: https://e-diccionesjustine-elp.net'la-vida-como-pre-texto-del-arte

Barrios, Fernando (2020a). "Jean Genet. A practice of saying. Life as a pretext of art". Available at: https://e-diccionesjustine-elp.net/la-vida-como-pre-texto-del-arte/

Barrios, Fernando (2020b). "Los afectos como política de lo subjetivo" (Affects as the politics of the subjective), in *ñacate.* Montevideo. Available at: http://www.revistanacate.com/articulos/de-los-afectos-como-politica-de-lo-subjetivo-fernando-barrios/

Barrios, Fernando (2020c). "On why olodumare is not god", in *Never we were Catholics. Orí Collective.* Available at: https://www.youtube.com/watch?v=GE3ne4M0ZfE

Barrios, Fernando and S. Filipini (2021). *De cuando Marx importunó a Lacan. A possible genealogy of the plus-de-jouir.* Montevideo: Escolios.

Bataille, Georges (1957). *La literatura y el mal.* Trans. Rafael Conte. Buenos Aires: Ediciones elaleph.com.

Bayard, Pierre (2008). *How to talk about books that have not been read.* Trans. Albert Galvanyr. Ed. Insurgentes. Available at: https://www.scribd.com'document'Bayard-Pierre-Pierre-How-To-Talk-About-The-Books.

Bayard, Pierre (2009). *Can literature be applied to psychoanalysis?* Trans. Viviana Ackerman. Buenos Aires: Paidós.

Beckett, Samuel. (2010). "Relatos", in *Texts for nothing.* Buenos Aires: Tusquets.

Benjamin, Walter (1985). *Capitalism as religion.* Trans. Enrique Foffani and Juan Antonio Ennis. Buenos Aires: Idihcs/unlp-conicet. Available at: http://ceiphistorica.com/wp-content/uploads/2016/05/Benjamin-Walter-El-capitalismo-como-religi%C3%B3n.pdf

Berlant, Laurent (2001). "Love, a queer feeling", in Tim Dean and Christopher Lane (eds.). *Homosexuality & Psychoanalysis*. Chicago.

Bersani, Leo (1998). *Homos*. Buenos Aires: Manantial.

Bersani, Leo (2011). *The Freudian body. Psychoanalysis and art*. Buenos Aires: El Cuenco de plata.

Bhabha, Homi J. (1994). *Les lieux de la culture. Une théorie post-coloniale*. Paris: Payot.

Bianchi, Soledad (2015). "Del neobarroco o la inestabilidad del taco alto: un neobarroco chilensis?". Available at: https://scielo.conicyt.cl/scielo.php?script=sci_arttext&pid=S0718-22952015000100018

Bonoris, Bruno J., and Muñoz, Pablo. (2021). "El cuerpo histérico y la sustancia gozante (The Hysterical Body and the Substance of Enjoyment)", in *Anuario de Investigaciones*, XXIV. Facultad de Psicología, Universidad de Buenos Aires, Secretaría de Investigaciones.

Bourlez, Fabrice (2018). *Queer psychanalyse. Clinique mineur et déconstructions du genre*. Paris: Hermann.

Braidotti, Rosi (2015). *Lo posthumano*. Barcelona: Gedisa.

Breuer, J. and Sigmund Freud (1987). "Katharina", in *Studies on Hysteria (1893–95). Complete Works*. Vol. 2. Buenos Aires: Amorrortu.

Butler, Judith (2006). *Precarious life. The power of mourning and violence*. Trans. Fermín Rodríguez. Buenos Aires-Barcelona: Paidós.

Butler, Judith (2007). *Gender in dispute. Feminism and the subversion of identity*. Buenos Aires: Paidós.

Butler, Judith (2015). "Transgenderism and the spirit of revolt". Available at: http://paroledequeer.blogspot.mx/2015/03/el-trangenero-y-el-espiritu-de-la.html

Cabral, Mauro and Gabriel Benzur. (2005). "When I say intersex. An introductory dialogue on intersexuality". Available at: www.scielo.br/scielo.php?script=sci_arttext&pid=S0104-83332005000100013

Califia, Patrick (2003). *Sex Changes Le mouvement transgenre, changer de sexe*. Paris: Epel.

Carvajal, Alberto (2021). "The performance of sexualities", in *e-dictions Justine de l'École lacanienne de psychanalyse*. Available at: https://e-diccionesjustine-elp.net/wp-content/uploads/2021/02/The-performance-of-sexualities.pdf

Chamoiseau, Patrick (1997). *Ecrire en pays domine*. Paris: Gallimard.

Cheng, François (2000). *Lacan and Chinese thought*. Available at: https://es.scribd.com/document/185023263/Lacan-y-El-Pensamiento-Chino-F-Cheng

Cherif, Zahar et al. (2019–2020). Available at: https://philosophie.univ-paris8.fr/cherif-zahar-Farah-irrera-Orazio-kisukidi-Nadia-Yala-renault-Matthieu-et

Comte, Auguste (1936). *Cours de philosophie positive*. Paris: Larousse.

Danowski, Deborah (2011). "Denialism. Holocaust, anthropocene. Studies in political theory". Available at: https://youtu.be/Yhy_U3Yyg4k

Davidson, Arnold I. (2011). "In praise of counter-conduct", in *History of the Human Sciences*, 24 (4), pp. 25–41.

De Aquino, Patricia (2000). "Le singulier pluriel du sexe. Contribution aux études de genre à partir des rituels afro- brésiliens du Candomblé", in *Journal des anthropologues*, 82–83, Anthropologie des sexualités, pp. 157–177.

de Brosses, Charles (1760). "Du culte des dieux fétiches ou Paralelle de l'Ancient religion de l'Egypte avec la religion actuelle de Nigrité". Available at: https://gallica.bnf.fr/ark:/12148/bpt6k106440f.texteImage

de Lauretis, Teresa (1991). "Teoría queer: sexualidades lesbianas y gays, una introducción", in *Differences: A Journal of Feminist Cultural Studies*, *3*(2), pp. iii–xvii

de Lauretis, Teresa (1993). "Eccentric subjects: Feminist theory and historical consciousness", in Maria C. Cangiamo and Lindsay DuBois (eds.). *From woman to gender, feminist theory, interpretation y práctica feministas en las ciencias sociales*. Buenos Aires: Centro Editor de América Latina.

de Lauretis, Teresa (1994). *The practice of love, lesbian sexuality and perverse desire. Desire*. Indiana University Press.
de Lauretis, Teresa (2014). *Conference at the interdisciplinary institute of gender studies (ffyl, uba)*. Buenos Aires: Carrera de Sociología (fsoc, uba) and Centro Cultural de la Cooperación Floreal Gorini.
de Rougemont, Denis (1945). *Love and the West*. Mexico: Ed. Leyenda.
Deleuze, Gilles and Felix Guattari (1998). *The anti-oedipus. Capitalism and schizophrenia*. Buenos Aires: Paidós.
Deleuze, Gilles and Felix Guattari (2002). *A thousand plateaus. Capitalismo y esquizofrenia*. Valencia: Pre textos.
Derrida, Jacques (1995). *Spectres of Marx. The state of debt, the work of mourning and the new international*. Madrid: Trotta.
Didi-Huberman, Georges (2016). *What a thrill, what a thrill?* Buenos Aires: Capital Intelectual.
Dieterleng, Germaine (ed.) (1993). *La notion de personne en Afrique noire*. Paris: L'Harmattan.
Dinshaw, Carolyn (1999). *Getting medieval: sexualities and communities, pre- and post-modern*. Durham, NC: Duke University Press.
Duras, Marguerite (1993). *Écrire*. Paris: Gallimard.
Dussel, Enrique (1993). *Marx's theological metaphors*. Madrid: Verbo divino. Available at: http://biblioteca.clacso.edu.ar/clacso/otros/20120522093839/2cap1.pdf
Edelman, Lee (2014). *No to the future. Queer theory and the death drive*. Barcelona: Egales.
Eribon, Didier (2001). *Reflexiones sobre la cuestión gay*. Editorial Anagrama.
Eribon, Didier (2004). *Una moral de lo minoritario: variaciones sobre un tema de Jean Genet*. Barcelona: Anagrama.
Eribon, Didier (2017). *Society as verdict. Classes, identities, trajectories*. Buenos Aires: El cuenco de plata.
Esquivel Flores, Aurea (2016). *Yaoi. Homoerotic pornography for women*. Available at: www.academia.edu/11850982/Yaoi._Homoerotic_pornography_for_women
Estrín (2002). "Lacan day by day". Available at: https://studylib.en/doc/8097721/diana-estr%C3%ADn-lacan-d%C3%ADa-por-d%C3%ADa---e-diciones-de-la-%C3%A9cole-
Etchegoyen, Horacio (2014). *The foundations of psychoanalytic technique*. Buenos Aires: Amorrortu. Available at: https://psicoanalisisonline.files.wordpress.com/2014/03/40641961-los-fundamentos-de-las-tecnica-psicoanalitica-etchegoyen-horacio.pdf
Fausto de Souza Coutinho, Juliana (2017). *A cosmopolítica dos animais*. PhD thesis in Philosophy, Department of Philosophy, PUC-Rio. Rio de Janeiro: Pontificia Universidade Católica do Rio de Janeiro.
Fernández, Aída (1960). "Confusion and acting out. Some aspects of the analysis of a homosexual patient". Available at: www.apuruguay.org/apurevista/1960/16887247196709O202.pdf
Fernández, Aída (1970). *Beauty, source of terror and fulfilment; A psychoanalytic approach to the conflict between ethical and aesthetic feeling in Aportes psicoanalíticos al estudio de la homosexualidad*. Montevideo: Oficina del Libro-aem.
Fisher, Mark (2018). *The ghosts of my life. Writings on depression, hauntology and lost futures*. Buenos Aires: Caja Negra Editora.
Flaksman, Clara (2018). *'De sangue' e 'de santo', o parentesco no Candomblé*. Rio de Janeiro: Federal University of Rio de Janeiro (ufrj) mana 24 (3), pp. 124–150. Disponible en: http://dx.doi.org/10.1590/1678-49442018v24n3p124
Fons, Virginia (2005). "Concepto de persona en África central". Available at: http://www.raco.cat/index.php/Orafrica/ article/download/135122/185302
Foucault, Michel (1967a). *History of madness*. Mexico: Fondo de Cultura Económica.

Foucault, Michel (1977b). *History of sexuality*. Vol. 1. The will to know. Madrid: Siglo xxi.
Foucault, Michel (1981). "De l'amitié comme mode de vie". Interview with R. de Ceccaty, J. Danet and Jean Le Bitoux, in Gai Pied, n. 25, April.
Foucault, Michel (1994). *Dits et écrits*. Vol. 3. Paris.
Foucault, Michel (2003). *History of sexuality*. Vol. 2. The use of pleasures. Madrid: Siglo xxi.
Freud, Sigmund (1986a). "Fetishism", in *Obras completas (1927–1931)*. Vol. 21. Buenos Aires: Amorrortu.
Freud, Sigmund (1986b). "Some psychical consequences of the anatomical difference of the sexes", in *Collected Works*. Vol. 19. Buenos Aires: Amorrortu.
Freud, Sigmund (1987). "Fragment of analysis of a case of hysteria (1905 [1901])", in *Collected Works*. Vol. 7. Buenos Aires: Amorrortu.
Freud, Sigmund (1988a). "Can laymen practice analysis? Dialogues with an impartial judge", in *Collected Works*. Vol. 20. Buenos Aires: Amorrortu.
Freud, Sigmund (1988b). "The future of an illusion", in *Obras completas*. Vol. 21. Buenos Aires: Amorrortu.
Freud, Sigmund (1989a). "El delirio y los sueños en la Gradiva de W Jensen", in *Obras completas*. Vol. 9. Buenos Aires: Amorrortu.
Freud, Sigmund (1989b). "On a particular type of object choice in man: contributions to the psychology of love (1910)", in *Collected Works*. Vol. 11. Buenos Aires: Amorrortu.
Freud, Sigmund (1989c). "On the psychogenesis of a case of female homosexuality (1920). homosexuality (1920)", in *Obras Completas*. Buenos Aires: Amorrortu.
Freud, Sigmund (1993). "Three essays on sexual theory (1905)", in *Obras Collected Works*. Vol. 7. Buenos Aires: Amorrortu.
Freud, Sigmund (2010). "Psychoanalytical remarks on a case of paranoia (Paranoid Dementia) autobiographically paranoia (Paranoid Dementia) described autobiographically", in *Collected Works*. Vol. 12. Buenos Aires: Amorrortu.
Garayalde, Nicolás (2018). "Literature and psychoanalysis: Towards a theory of reading". Available at: https://www.academia.edu/38362156
Rubin, Gayle (1975). "The traffic in women: Notes on the 'political economy' of sex", in Rayna Reiter (ed.). *Toward an anthropology of women*. New York: Monthly Review Press
Genet, Jean (1947). *Pompas fúnebres*. Trans. María Teresa Gallego and María Isabel Reverte. Madrid: Debate.
Genet, Jean (1976). *Diary of the thief.* Trans. Ma. Teresa Gallego and Isabel Reverte. Barcelona: Planeta.
Genet, Jean (2003). *Querelle de Brest*. Trans. Felicitas Sánchez Mediero and Santiago Roncagliolo. Madrid: Odisea.
Gerber, Daniel (2012). *"Una (necesaria) crítica de la noción de género desde el psicoanálisis" (A (necessary) critique of the notion of gender from psychoanalysis)*. Mexico: Círculo Psicoanalítico Mexicano, 23 November. Available at: https://youtu.be/VSg_8Pa97wo
Goldman, Marcio (1985). "A construção ritual da pessoa: a possessão no Candomblé", in *Religião e Sociedade*, 12 (1), August, pp. 22–54.
Guzmán, Manolo (1997). "Pa la Escuelita con mucho cuidao y por la orillita": A Journey Through theContested Terrains of the Nation and Sexual Orientation. In Frances Negrón-Muntaner & Ramón Grosfoguel (Eds.), *Puerto Rican Jam: Rethinking Colonialism and Nationalism*. pp. 209–228. Minneapolis: University of Minnesota Press.
Halberstam, Judith (2008). *Masculinidad femenina*. Barcelona: Egales.
Halberstam, Judith (2015). "The antisocial turn in queer studies", in *The* queer *body. queer. Subverting heteronormativity*. Buenos Aires: Letra Viva and Lecol.
Halperin, David (2000). *San Foucault*. Edelp, Cuadernos de Litoral.
Halperin, David (2015). *L'Art d'être gai*. Paris: EPEL.
Halperin, David (2019). "Queer love". Available at: https://e-diccionesjustine-elp.net/amor-queer-un-texto-de-david-halperin-introduction-and-commentary-by-rafael-perez-y-martin-perez/

Haraway, Donna (1991). "A Cyborg Manifesto: Science, Technology, and SocialistFeminism in the Late Twentieth Century", in Simians, Cyborgs and Women: The Reinvention of Nature. New York: Routledge.
Haraway, Donna (2018). "Sympoiesis, CF, multispecies muddles", in *Nomadic Divans. Embrollos e historias*. Vol. 5. Revista de la école lacanienne de psychanalyse. Córdoba.
Haraway, Donna (2019a). "When species meet: Introductions", in *Tábula rasa*, 31, pp. 23–75. Available at: www.revistatabularasa.org'number31'when-the-species-meets
Haraway, Donna (2019b). *Getting on with the problem. Generating kinship in the Chthuluceno*. Trans. Helen Torres. Bilbao: Consonni.
Hart, Lynda (1998). *The sadomasochistic performance. Between body andflesh*. Paris: Epel.
Heidegger, Martin (1987). *On the way to speech*. Available at: https://www.academia.edu/15269284/de_camino_al_habla_martin_heidegger
Hernández, Felisberto (2002a). "Diary of the scoundrel", in *Obras completas*. Vol. 3. Montevideo: Arca.
Hernández, Felisberto (2002b). "Fulano de tal", in *Obras Completas*. Vol. 1. Montevideo: Arca, Mdeo.
Hernández, Felisberto (2002c). "Sobre Literatura", in *Obras Completas*. Vol. 3. Montevideo: Arca.
Hernández, Manuel (2013). "La rotura y la vergüenza", in *Historia del psicoanálisis*. Mexico: Instituto del Derecho de Asilo-Museo de León Trosky.
Hocquenghem, Guy (2009). *Homosexual desire. Anal terror*. Spain: Melusina.
Hocquenghem, Guy (2020). "The future belongs to the couple. El estar-de-a-dos, totalitarian form of modernity", in *ñacate*. Available at: http://www.revistanacate.com/fronteras/el-futuro-belongs-to-the-couple-being-of-two-totalitarian-form-of-modernity-guy-hocquenghem/
Lacan, Jacques (1966). *On structure as mixture. of otherness, a sine qua non condition of absolutely any subject*. Trans. Leonel Sánchez Trapani. Baltimore. Available at: http://www.bibliopsi.org/docs/lacan/Lacan-Acerca-de-la-estructura-como-mixtura-de-una-otredad-1966.pdf
Lacan, Jacques (1967). "Brief address to psychiatrists". Available at: https://www.lacanterafreudiana.com.ar/2.5.1.12%20%20%20brief%20discurso%20A%20los%20psiquiatras,%201967.pdf
Lacan, Jacques (1971). "Lituraterre", in *Revista Litératture*. Vol. 3. Trans. Ricardo Rodríguez Ponte. Available at: https://elpsicoanalistalector.blogspot.com/2012/04/jacques-lacan-lituraterre-1971-version.html
Lacan, Jacques (1972). "Lecture in Louvain". Available at: https://youtu.be/-HBnLAK4_Cc
Lacan, Jacques (1977). "Preface to the English edition of Seminar xi". Available at: http://elpsicoanalistalector.blogspot.com/2009/04/jacques-lacan-preface-the-edition.html
Lacan, Jacques (1984a). "El atolondradradicho", in *Ornicar?*, Vol. 1. Buenos Aires: Paidós Biblioteca Freudiana.
Lacan, Jacques (1984b). "Intervention on transference", in *Writings 1*. Mexico: Siglo xxi.
Lacan, Jacques (1984c). *Seminar 3 Las Psicosis (1955–56)*. Buenos Aires: Paidós.
Lacan, Jacques (1985). "Variants of the type-cure", in *Writings 1*. Mexico, Siglo xxi.
Lacan, Jacques (1986). *Seminar 11 The four fundamental concepts of psychoanalysis (1964)*. Buenos Aires: Paidós.
Lacan, Jacques (1992). *Seminar 17 The reverse side of psychoanalysis (1969–70)*. Buenos Aires: Paidós.
Lacan, Jacques (1993). *Psychoanalysis radio & television*. Trans. and Notes by Oscar Masotta and Orlando Gimeno-Grendi. Barcelona: Anagrama.
Lacan, Jacques (1994). *Seminar 4 The object relation (1957)*. Buenos Aires: Paidós.
Lacan, Jacques (2001). "Homenaje a Marguerite Duras, del arrebato de Lol. V Stein (1965)", in *Autres écrits*. Paris: du Seuil.

Lacan, Jacques (2003–2004). *L ínsu que sait de l úne bévue s áile à mourre (1976–1977)*. Trans. Graciela Leguizamón, María del Carmen Melegatti and Rafael Perez. Available at: www.ecole-lacanienne.net/bibliotheque
Lacan, Jacques (2006a). *On paranoid psychosis in its relation to personality (1932)*. Mexico: Siglo xxi.
Lacan, Jacques (2006b). *Seminar 10 La angustia (1962–63)*. Buenos Aires: Paidós.
Lacan, Jacques (2006c). *Seminar 23 The sinthome (1975–76)*. Buenos Aires: Paidós.
Lacan, Jacques (2007). *Seminar L'etourdit*. Available at: http://staferla.free.fr/Lacan/L'etourdit.pdf
Lacan, Jacques (2008a). *Seminar 16 From an other to the other (1968–69)*. Buenos Aires: Paidós.
Lacan, Jacques (2008b). *Seminar 20 Even (1972–73)*. Buenos Aires: Paidós.
Lacan, Jacques (2012a). "Nota italiana", in *Otros escritos*. Buenos Aires: Paidós.
Lacan, Jacques (2012b). "Televisión (1972)", in *Otros escritos*. Buenos Aires: Paidós.
Lacan, Jacques (2012c). *The seminar book 19 or worse (1971–72)*. Buenos Aires: Paidós.
Lacan, Jacques and Vladimir Granoff (2015). "Fetishism: The symbolic, the imaginary and the real". Available at: https:// www.acheronta.org/lacan/fetichismo.htm
Latour, Bruno (2007). *We were never modern. Ensayo de Antropología simétrica*. Buenos Aires: Siglo xxi.
Leff, Gloria (2021). *Lo oculto, verdad indómita. Freud, István Hollos . . . and others*. Mexico: Epeele. École lacanienne de psychanalyse.
Lemebel, Pedro (1997). "Manifiesto", in *Loco afán, crónicas de sidario*. Santiago de Chile, Lom.
Lemebel, Pedro (2000). *Loco afán. Crónicas de sidario*. Barcelona.
Lemebel, Pedro (2013). *Little man. Crónicas escogidas 1989–2012*. Chile: UDP.
Lemebel, Pedro (2018). *I don't have friends, I have loves. Extracts from interviews*. Ed Alchemy.
Liu, Wen (2020). "Sentir abatido, regresivo y maquínico: Teoría queer y el giro afectivo.", in *Athenea Digital 20*(2), e2321.
Lockhart, Washington (1991). *Felisberto Hernández, una biografía literaria*. Montevideo: Arca.
Lorde, A. (2003). *La hermana, la extranjera. Articles and conferences (1979)*. Trans. María Corniero. Madrid: Horas y horas.
Louis, Édouard (2019). *To end with Eddy Bellegueule*. Barcelona: Salamandra.
Love, Heather (2007). *Feeling backward. Loss and the politics of queer history*. Cambridge and London: Harvard University Press.
Maristany, José (2008). "A Latin American queer theory? Poststructuralism and identity politics in Lemebel". Available at: https://lecturesdugenrefr.files.wordpress.com/2019/03/maristany.pdf
Márquez, Nicolás and Agustín Lage (2016). *El libro negro de la nueva izquierda. Gender ideology or cultural subversion*. Buenos Aires: Pesur.
Marx, Karl (1968). *Manuscritos económicos políticos de 1844*. Madrid: Alianza.
Marx, Karl (2001). "The commodity", in *Capital: Critique of political economy*. Barcelona: Orbis.
Medina, Cuauhtémoc. (2010). *Sur, sur, sur, sur, sur*. Mexico: PAC-SITAC.
Melville, Herman (1854). *The enchanted women*. Available at: Titivillus ePub base r1.2; 2017 https://pdfcoffee.com/melville-herman-las-enchanted-3-pdf-free.html
Melville, Herman (2013). *Billy Bud, sailor*. Available at: http://www.librosdearena.es/Biblioteca_pdf/melville_herman_Billy%20Buddmarinero.pdf
Michel, Foucault (1996). *La vida de los hombres infames*. Editorial Altamira, Calle 49 N° 540, La Plata, Argentina
Mignolo, Walter (2007). *The idea of Latin America*. Barcelona: Gedisa.

Miller, Gérard (2011). "Rendez- vous chez Lacan". Available at: https://www.youtube.com/watch?v=9Xvfb8mpp18
Miller, Jacques A. (2021). "Docile au trans". Available at: https://laregledujeu.org/2021/04/22/37014/transsexuel- docile-au-trans/
Monsivais, Carlos (2007). "Pedro Lemebel. Del barroco desclosetado". Available at: www.revistadelauniversidad.unam.mx/4207/pdfs/5-12.pdf
Morton, Timothy (2018). *Hyperobjects. Philosophy and ecology after the end of the world.* Buenos Aires: Adriana Hidalgo.
Motta, C. (2013). *The films Lacan saw and applied to psychoanalysis*. Buenos Aires: Paidós.
Mudimbe, Valentin-Y. (1988). *The invention of Africa.* Bloomington-Indianapolis-London, Indiana: University Press – James Currey.
Muñoz, José Esteban (1999). *Disidentifications. queers of color and the performance of politics cultural studies of the Americas*. Vol. 2. University of Minnesota Press.
Nadaud, Stéphane (2017). *Subjective fragments*. Buenos Aires: Cactus.
Oyewumi, Oyeronké (2017). *The invention of women. An African perspective on Western discourses of gender*. Bogotá: Editorial en la frontera.
Pardo, José Luis (2000). "Bartleby o de la humanidad. Universidad Complutense de Madrid". Available at: http://www.academia.edu/887446/Bartleby_o_de_la_humanidad?auto=download
Pereda, Alberto (1968). "Aspects of male homosexual acting-out", in *Revista Uruguaya de Psicoanálisis*., 10, pp. 267–274.
Perlongher, Néstor (1980). *Why we will be so beautiful in Austria-Hungary*. Buenos Aires: Tierra Baldía.
Perlongher, Néstor (1991). *Antropología del éxtasis*. Reprint, Buenos Aires: Editorial Urania, 2021.Platero, Raquel (Lucas) (2014). *Interview with Judith Halberstam*. Available at: paroledequeer.blogspot.com
Preciado, Beatriz (2008). *Testo yonqui*. Madrid: Espasa Escalpe.
Preciado, Beatriz (2009). "La invención del género, o el tecnocordero que devours the wolves. Biopolítica del Género", in *Conversaciones Feministas, Biopolítica*. Buenos Aires: Ají de pollo.
Preciado, Beatriz (2014a). Available at: https://www.youtube.com/watch?v=vtbGyKqYtTk
Preciado, Beatriz (2014b). *Interview with Paul B. Preciado: Postporno/Dissident Excitement*. Available at: paroledequeer.blogspot.com/2014/01/entrevista-con-beatriz-preciado.html
Preciado, Beatriz (2015a). *The death of the clinic? Living and resisting in the neoliberal condition*. Bocabulvaria ediciones.
Preciado, Paul B. (2015b). "Pearls and scars for Pedro Lemebel". Available at: paroledequeer.blogspot.com/2015/01/perlas-y-cicatrices-para-pedro-lemebel.html
Preciado, Paul B. (2019a). *A flat in Uranus. Chronicles of the crossroads*. Barcelona: Anagrama.
Preciado, Paul B. (2019b). *Intervention at the 49th Conference of the École de la Cause Freudienne women in psychoanalysis*. Paris, 17 November.
Preciado, Paul B. (2015). "Happy Valentine". Available at: http://paroledequeer.blogspot.com/2015/02/happy-valentine-por-paul-b-preciado.html
Reitter, Jorge N. (2019). *Oedipo gay. Heteronormativity and psychoanalysis*. Buenos Aires: Letra Viva.
Rieder, Inés and Diana Voigt (2004). *Sidonie Csillag. Freud's young homosexual*. Buenos Aires: El cuenco de plata.
Rivat, Mathieu and Aurélien Berland (2016). "Discussion with Isabelle Stengers on neopagan witches and modern science", in *Divanes nomades. Traces and flashes in the margins*. Vol. 3. Córdoba.
Rivera Cusicanqui, Silvia (2018). *A Ch'ixi world is possible*. Buenos Aires: Tinta Limón.

Rodrigues, Luis (2018). *Pedagogía das encruzilhadas*. Available at: https://doi.org/10.12957/periferia.2018.31504
Roughton, R (2001a).Cuatro hombres en tratamiento: una perspectiva en evolución sobre la homosexualidad y la bisexualidad". *J Am Psychoanal Assoc* 49, 1187–217
Rubin, Gayle (1975). "The traffic in women: Notes on the 'political economy' of sex", in Rayna Reiter (ed.). *Toward an anthropology of women*. New York: Monthly Review Press.
Rubino, Atilio (1975). "The queer monster in the rocky horror picture show. Sexuality, gender and parody camp in horror cinema". Available at: www.archivosdelafilmoteca.com
Saez, Javier (2015). *El amor es heterosexual. The queer body. Subvertir la heteronormatividad*. Buenos Aires: Letra Viva and Lecol.
Sahlins, Marshall (2011). "What kinship is (part one)", in *Journal of the Royal Anthropological Institute*, 17, pp. 2–29.
Sartre, Jean Paul (1967). *Saint Genet, comedian and martyr*. Trans. Luis Echávarri. Buenos Aires: Losada.
Saxe, Facundo (2018). "La trampa mortal: derivas maricas de la disidencia disidencia sexual en la producción de conocimiento científico al recuerdo infantil de un beso", in *Etcétera*. Revista Del Área De Ciencias Sociales Del CIFFyH. Vol. 3. Córdoba: UNC. Available at: https://revistas.unc.edu.ar/index.php/etcetera/article/view/22591
Schroeder, Damian (2010). "*Dialogues with the works La apropiación de la belleza by Gladys Franco and Correspondencias entre Silvia Bleichmar y Hanif Kureishi* by Daniel Moreira". Available at: www.apuruguay.org/apurevista/2010/16887247201111317.pdf
Segato, Rita (2015). "El Edipo brasilero: la doble negación de género y raza", in *La crítica de la colonialidad en ocho ensayos y una antropología por demanda*. Buenos Aires: Prometeo.
Silvestri, Leonor (2020). "Heterocapitalism and madness". Available at: https://www.youtube.com/watch?v=MpEZ-2ky9HM
Solana, Mariela (2016). "Reflexiones sobre el giro afectivo en historia queer", in *Mora*, Revista del Instituto Interdisciplinario de Estudios de Género. Vol. 22, n. 1. Buenos Aires: Facultad de Filosofía y Letras, Universidad de Buenos Aires, June.
Spivac, Gayatri (2003). "Can the subaltern speak?" Available at: www.memoria.fahce.unlp.edu.ar/art_revistas/pr.2732/pr.2732.pdf
Sprinkle, Annie (2017). "Nature is your lover, not your mother: Meet ecosexual Pioneer". Available at: https://www.theguardian.com'Lifestyle'Women
Stengers, Isabelle (2009). *In times of catastrophe. How surviving the coming barbarism*. Ned Editions. Available at: https://www.academia.edu/40320616/En_tiempos_de_catastrofes_C%C3%B3mo_resistir_a_a_la_barbarie_que_viene_Isabelle_Stengers
Strongman, Roberto (2019). "Queering black atlantics religions. Transcorporeality", in *Candomble, Santeria and Voudou*. Durham and London: Duke University Press.
Tin, Louis-Georges (2012). *The invention of heterosexual culture*. Buenos Aires: El Cuenco de plata.
Tiqqun (1999). *Of economics considered as black magic. A metaphysical critique*. Available at: https://tiqqunim.blogspot.com/2013/02/de-la-economia-considerada-como-como-magia.html
Vasallo, Sara (2015). "The atheism of Jacques Lacan". Available at: www.elsigma.com/filosofia/el-ateismo-de-j-lacan/12996
Vila-Matas, Enrique (2013). *Autobiography*. Available at: http://www.enriquevilamatas.com/autobiografia.html
Vila-Matas, Enrique (2015). *Bartleby y compañía*. Madrid: Seix Barral.
Viltard, Mayette (2021). "Los públicos de Freud", in *Me cayó el veinte*, 40.
Viveiros de Castro, Eduardo and Deborah Danowski (2019). *Is there a world to come? Essay on fears and ends*. Buenos Aires: Caja Negra.
Vives, Juan (2014). "Can homosexuals practice psychoanalysis?" Available at: fepal.org/images/./can_homosexuals_practice_psychoanalysis.pdf

Weber, Max (2004). *La ética protestante y el espíritu del capitalismo*. Mexico: Premia Editora.
Wilde, Oscar (2016). *De profundis*. Montevideo: Penguin.
Willful Subjects (2014). Durham and London: Duke University Press.
Wittig, Monique (2006). *El pensamiento heterosexual y otros ensayos*. Barcelona: Egales.

Index

For Product Safety Concerns and Information please contact our EU representative GPSR@taylorandfrancis.com
Taylor & Francis Verlag GmbH, Kaufingerstraße 24, 80331 München, Germany

www.ingramcontent.com/pod-product-compliance
Ingram Content Group UK Ltd.
Pitfield, Milton Keynes, MK11 3LW, UK
UKHW020002200926
475702UK00015B/2432

* 9 7 8 1 0 4 1 1 9 1 4 9 0 *